DERMATOLOGY - LABORATORY AND CLINICAL RESEARCH

ATOPIC DERMATITIS

A REVIEW FOR THE PRIMARY CARE PHYSICIAN

DERMATOLOGY - LABORATORY AND CLINICAL RESEARCH

Additional books in this series can be found on Nova's website under the Series tab.

Additional E-books in this series can be found on Nova's website under the E-books tab.

PUBLIC HEALTH IN THE 21ST CENTURY

Additional books in this series can be found on Nova's website under the Series tab.

Additional E-books in this series can be found on Nova's website under the E-books tab.

DERMATOLOGY - LABORATORY AND CLINICAL RESEARCH

ATOPIC DERMATITIS

A REVIEW FOR THE PRIMARY CARE PHYSICIAN

ALEXANDER K. C. LEUNG
AND
KAM LUN E. HON

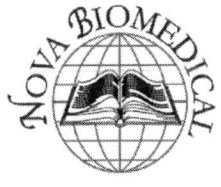

Nova Science Publishers, Inc.
New York

Copyright © 2012 by Nova Science Publishers, Inc.

All rights reserved. No part of this book may be reproduced, stored in a retrieval system or transmitted in any form or by any means: electronic, electrostatic, magnetic, tape, mechanical photocopying, recording or otherwise without the written permission of the Publisher.

For permission to use material from this book please contact us:
Telephone 631-231-7269; Fax 631-231-8175
Web Site: http://www.novapublishers.com

NOTICE TO THE READER

The Publisher has taken reasonable care in the preparation of this book, but makes no expressed or implied warranty of any kind and assumes no responsibility for any errors or omissions. No liability is assumed for incidental or consequential damages in connection with or arising out of information contained in this book. The Publisher shall not be liable for any special, consequential, or exemplary damages resulting, in whole or in part, from the readers' use of, or reliance upon, this material. Any parts of this book based on government reports are so indicated and copyright is claimed for those parts to the extent applicable to compilations of such works.

Independent verification should be sought for any data, advice or recommendations contained in this book. In addition, no responsibility is assumed by the publisher for any injury and/or damage to persons or property arising from any methods, products, instructions, ideas or otherwise contained in this publication.

This publication is designed to provide accurate and authoritative information with regard to the subject matter covered herein. It is sold with the clear understanding that the Publisher is not engaged in rendering legal or any other professional services. If legal or any other expert assistance is required, the services of a competent person should be sought. FROM A DECLARATION OF PARTICIPANTS JOINTLY ADOPTED BY A COMMITTEE OF THE AMERICAN BAR ASSOCIATION AND A COMMITTEE OF PUBLISHERS.

Additional color graphics may be available in the e-book version of this book.

Library of Congress Cataloging-in-Publication Data

Leung, Alexander K. C.
 Atopic dermatitis : a review for the primary care physician / Alexander K.C. Leung, Kam Lun E. Hon.
     p. ; cm.
 Includes bibliographical references and index.
 ISBN 978-1-61324-540-8 (softcover)
 1. Atopic dermatitis. I. Hon, K. L. E. (Kam Lun Ellis) II. Title.
 [DNLM: 1. Dermatitis, Atopic. 2. Primary Health Care--methods. WR 160]
 RL243.L48 2010
 616.5'1--dc23
                                                                          2011014220

Published by Nova Science Publishers, Inc. † New York

Contents

Preface		vii
Chapter I	Introduction	1
Chapter II	Epidemiology	3
Chapter III	Pathogenesis and Etiology	5
Chapter IV	Immunopathology	15
Chapter V	Clincial Manifestations	17
Chapter VI	Diagnosis	21
Chapter VII	Assessment of Severity and Psychosocial Impact	25
Chapter VIII	Differential Diagnosis	29
Chapter IX	Complications	31
Chapter X	Diagnostic Testing	35
Chapter XI	Management	39
Chapter XII	Prognosis	69
Chapter XIII	Conclusion	71
References		73
Index		105

Preface

Atopic dermatitis is a chronically relapsing dermatosis characterized by pruritus, erythema, vesiculation, papulation, exudation, excoriation, crusting, scaling, and sometimes lichenification.Atopic dermatitis affects 10 to 20% of school-aged children. The prevalence of atopic dermatitis has increased two- to three folds over the past three decades in industrialized countries and there is evidence to suggest that this prevalence is increasing.The increase in prevalence may be due to increased access to medical care, improved recognition, better epidemiological reporting, or increased environmental allergens due to industrialization and pollution. The pathogenesis of atopic dermatitis involves complex interactions between susceptible genes, immunological factors, skin barrier defects, infections, neuroendocrine factors, and environmental factors. Two forms of atopic dermatitis have been delineated: an extrinsic form associated with IgE-mediated sensitization involving 70 to 80% of patients and an intrinsic form without IgE-mediated sensitization involving 20 to 30% of the patients.

Approximately 60% of children with atopic dermatitis manifest the disease by the first year of life and an additional 30% before the age of 5 years. The clinical manifestations vary with age and may differ during the course of disease. In infants, the eruption often affects the face and scalp, although the extensor surfaces of the extremities and the trunk may also be affected. In older children and adolescents, the neck and antecubital and popliteal fossae usually display the eruption. In adults, eczematous involvement of the neck, hands, and flexures are typical findings and atopic dermatitis may present as dyshidrotic eruptions. Atopic lesions are classified as acute, subacute, or chronic and are usually symmetrical. Acute lesions are intensely pruritic, erythematous papules, papulovesicles, or weeping lesions. Subacute lesions are erythematous scaling papules or excoriated plaques. Chronic lesions are characterized by prominent scaling, excoriations, and lichenification in classically affected body areas. There is no central clearing. Exacerbations and remissions are common and to be expected.

A number of scoring systems have been developed for the assessment of disease severity in children with atopic dermatitis. The SCORing of Atopic Dermatitis (SCORAD) system, Eczema Area and Severity Index (EASI) system, and the Nottingham Eczema Severity Score (NESS) system are user-friendly, relatively reliable, and in popular use. These systems generate quantifiable data that are amenable to analysis. The choice of which scale to use is a matter of personal preference. A number of indices have been designed to measure the impact of the disease on the quality of life of affected children and the parents. Although some studies have shown a positive correlation between children's and parents' quality of life and disease severity on cross-sectional and over-time observation, there is not necessarily a direct relation between the severity of atopic dermatitis and its impact on quality of life. The quality of life measurement provides additional information to the objective clinical scoring systems.Although the scoring systems for assessment of disease severity and psychosocial impact have often been used to assess outcomes in clinical trials, they are rarely used in clinical practice.

Secondary bacterial infection, most commonly with *Staphylococcus aureus*, is the main complication of atopic dermatitis.Eczema herpeticum caused by herpes simplex virus is a potentially dangerous complication.Atopic dermatitis can be quite uncomfortable and distressing to patients because of the associated pruritus and unsightly lesions. Because of associated emotional stress and sleep disruption, the impact on the quality of life of patients and families can be significant. Atopic dermatitis is an initiating factor in the atopic march as more than 50% of patients with atopic dermatitis subsequently develop asthma or allergic rhinitis.

Avoidance of triggering factors, optimal skin care, and topical corticosteroids are the mainstay of therapy for atopic dermatitis.Topical immunomodulators (tacrolimus and pimecrolimus) are beneficial and safe for adults and children over 2 years of age.Topical immunomodulators represent a major new alternative to chronic corticosteroid use.

Alexander K.C. Leung
MBBS, FRCPC, FRCP (UK & Irel), FRCPCH, FAAP,
Clinical Professor of Pediatrics, The University of Calgary,
Pediatric Consultant,
Alberta Children's Hospital,
Calgary, Alberta, Canada T2M 0H5
Email: aleung@ucalgary.ca

Kam Lun E. Hon
MD, MBBS, FAAP, FCCM,
Professor of Pediatrics,The Chinese University of Hong Kong,
Prince of Wales Hospital,
Shatin, Hong Kong SAR, China

Chapter I

Introduction

Atopic dermatitis is a chronically relapsing dermatosis characterized by pruritus, erythema, vesiculation, papulation, exudation, excoriation, crusting, scaling, and sometimes lichenification [1-3]. The word *atopic* comes from the Greek word *atopos*, meaning "strange" or "unusual". Atopic eczema is synonymous with atopic dermatitis. The word *eczema* is derived from the Greek word *ekzema*, meaning "erupt" or "boil over". Atopic dermatitis is an "itch that rashes".

The prevalence of atopic dermatitis has increased two- to three folds over the past three decades in industrialized countries and there is evidence to suggest that this prevalence is increasing [4-7]. The increase in prevalence may be due to increased access to medical care, improved recognition, better epidemiological reporting, or increased environmental allergens due to industrialization and pollution [8]. Two forms of atopic dermatitis have been delineated: an extrinsic form associated with IgE-mediated sensitization involving 70 to 80% of patients and an intrinsic form without IgE-mediated sensitization involving 20 to 30% of the patients [6,9]. The latter is often referred to as atopiform dermatitis [10]. Children with extrinsic atopic dermatitis exhibit allergen-specific IgE to aeroallergens and food, positive skin prick reaction, and a positive history of asthma and allergic rhinitis [11]. Atopic dermatitis most often presents in infancy or early childhood [1-3]. It is an initiating factor in the atopic march as more than 50% of patients with atopic dermatitis subsequently develop asthma or allergic rhinitis [12,13]. Both forms have associated eosinophilia [14]. Atopic dermatitis is frustrating to both patients and caregivers. The pruritus can be intractable and the disease has important physical and psychological implications. Because of associated emotional stress and sleep disruption, the impact on the quality of life of patients and families can be significant. Although there is no cure, control is possible in most patients with optimal skin care, pharmacotherapy, and adherence to preventive measures.

Chapter II

Epidemiology

Atopic dermatitis affects 10 to 20% of children and 1 to 3% of adults in the United States and Europe [15-21]. The prevalence is increasing, especially in developing countries [22]. The actual incidence of atopic dermatitis is hard to estimate because most studies have examined point prevalence [23]. The prevalence is higher in developed countries and urban areas, and in populations that move from an area of low to high prevalence, probably due to modifications in the lifestyle and environment [4,19,23]. Atopic dermatitis occurs more frequently in temperate rather than tropical areas [24]. The condition is also more prevalent in children that belong to advantaged socioeconomic classes, smaller family sizes, and families with overzealous hygiene [4,20,25]. Children who have more infections in infancy tend to be less frequently affected [26]. There is no significant difference in prevalence between preterm and term children [27]. There is a lack of correlation between body mass index and atopic dermatitis [20,28,29].

Approximately 30 to 50% of children with one affected parent and 50 to 80% with two affected parents develop the disorder [30]. There is a higher risk associated with maternal rather than paternal atopy [31-33]. The condition is slightly more common in females than males with a female to male ratio of 1.5:1 [34]. Female patients with atopic dermatitis often experience worsening of cutaneous symptoms associated with their pregnancy or menstrual cycle [35].

Chapter III

Pathogenesis and Etiology

The pathogenesis of atopic dermatitis involves complex interactions between susceptible genes, immunological factors, skin barrier defects, infections, neuroendocrine factors, and environmental factors [1,17,36]. Patients may exhibit IgE-mediated sensitization due to external antigens or intrinsic sensitization, without IgE-mediated sensitization [37].

There is a strong genetic predisposition to atopic dermatitis, as evidenced by the familial nature of the disease and the high concordance in monozygotic twins [1-3]. Twin studies have shown much higher disease concordance for monozygotic twins (72 to 86%) when compared with dizygotic twins (15 to 23%), suggesting the role of genetic factor in the pathogenesis of atopic dermatitis [4,38,39]. Based on linkage genes analysis studies and candidate gene studies, numerous gene loci have been mapped on different chromosomes including, among others, 1q21, 3p24-26, 3q14, 3q21, 4p14-15, 5q31-33, 11q13, 13q14, 14q11, 17q25, 18q11-12, and 20p [33,40,41].

It has been shown that loss-of-function mutations in the filaggrin (*FLG*) gene results in increased permeability of the skin to proteins, thereby increasing the risk of allergic sensitization [42]. These gene defects thus predispose to extrinsic, but not intrinsic atopic dermatitis [9,31,43-45]. A recent systematic review and meta-analysis found that *FLG* gene defects are associated with a substantial increased risk of atopic dermatitis with an odds ratio of 1.99 (95% confidence interval: 1.72 to 2.31) in the family studies and an odds ratio of 4.78 (95% confidence interval: 3.31 to 6.92) in the case control studies [46]. Another systematic review by Rodríguez et al confirmed the strong and consistent association between *FLG* mutations and atopic dermatitis in 24 case-control and family studies (odds ratio:

3.12; 95% confidence interval: 2.57 to 3.79) and even stronger associations with dermatologist-diagnosed atopic dermatitis (odds ratio: 4.24; 95% confidence interval: 3.09 to 5.81) and moderate to severe cases of atopic dermatitis (odds ratio: 5.16; 95% confidence interval: 3.92 to 6.8)[47]. *FLG* is located on chromosome 1q21 [10,48]. Mutations in the *FLG* gene are present in approximately 10 to 50% of patients with atopic dermatitis [49].Five *FLG* null mutations, namely R501X, 2282del4, R2447X, S2554X, and S2889Xare some of the more popular mutations identified in Caucasian and Japanese populations[50].However, 2282del4, R2447X, S2554X and S2889X mutations were not found in a study among Cantonese Chinese [50].Heterozygous carriage of R501X was only found in four male patients, and associated with long-term disease severity.*FLG* mutations that are prevalent in Caucasian and other Asian populations are rarely found in our seriesof patients in Hong Kong[50].

Atopic dermatitis involves defective cell-mediated immunity related, in part, to an imbalance in two subsets of CD4- T-cells that creates a predominance of T-memory cells in the T-helper 2 pathways and preferential apoptosis of interferon-gamma producing T-helper 1 memory and effector T-cells [3,4]. T-helper 2 cells express a set of cytokines (interleukin-4, -5, -6, -10, and -13) [51-53]. Cytokines are released from cells in the skin, attracting other inflammatory cells and producing other inflammatory mediators and reactions. These cytokines stimulate the proliferation and differentiation of B-lymphocytes, upregulate the expression of adhesion molecules on endothelial cells, and contribute to the hypereosinophilia, high serum IgE levels, sustained cutaneous inflammation, histamine release, and pruritus characteristic of the atopic dermatitis [4,24,51,53]. Compared with extrinsic atopic dermatitis, the intrinsic form is associated with lower expression of interleukin-4, -5, and -13 and higher expression of interferon-γ [6,9]. Maintenance of chronic inflammation is associated with predominance of interleukin-5 and -12 expression and eosinophils [24].

Impairment of the barrier function of the skin is an important etiologic factor in the pathogenesis of extrinsic, but not intrinsic, atopic dermatitis [9,53]. The skin has two barrier structures, namely, the stratum corneum and tight junctions [54]. The stratum corneum acts as a barrier in preventing water loss from the skin and in protecting the skin from intrusion by irritants and micro-organisms [55]. In patients with atopic dermatitis, the stratum corneum can be dysfunctional as a result of defects in FLG, reduced content of ceramides, and physical trauma [54]. FLG, an epidermal barrier protein, plays an important role in the barrier function of the skin [43,56,57]. Tight junctions reside immediately below the stratum corneum and regulate the selective permeability of the paracellular pathway [54]. Some authors have speculated thattight junctions might regulate the lipid components found in the stratum corneum [58,59]. The transepidermal water loss in atopic dermatitis lesions is significantly greater as compared with non-lesional atopic dermatitis skin and healthy skin [54,60]. It has been shown that the transepidermal water loss in atopic dermatitis lesions is not attributable to *FLG* mutations [54,61,62]. Rather, the transepidermal water loss results from a dysfunction of keratinocyte tight junctions [62].

FLG protein is present in the granular layers of the epidermis and the keratohyalin granules in the granular layers are predominantly composed of profilaggrin [63]. FLG proteins aggregate the keratin cytoskeleton system to form a dense protein-lipid matrix that is cross-linked by transglutaminases to form the cornified cell envelope [43,63]. The latter prevents epidermal water loss and impedes the entry of allergens, infectious agents, and chemicals [36,43]. In addition, degradation products of FLG such as amino acids contribute to the composition of natural moisturizing factor in the stratum corneum [64]. It is believed that defective epidermal function is related to the down-regulation of the *FLG* gene and reduced ceramide levels [17].

There is evidence that skin barrier dysfunction precedes skin inflammation and clinical manifestations of atopic dermatitis [56]. Flohr et al evaluated 88 infants and analyzed them for both clinical evidence of skin inflammation and barrier dysfunction at 3 months of age [56]. Twenty nine (33%) of these children had clinical evidence of atopic dermatitis. The authors found that *FLG* mutation carriers were more likely to have atopic dermatitis than non-carriers. They also found that *FLG* mutation carriers had worsened skin barrier function, drier skin, and increased transepidermal water loss compared with non-carriers. The observation that transepidermal water loss is elevated in unaffected *FLG* mutation carriers suggests that skin barrier impairment precedes clinical atopic dermatitis [56].

A reduced content of ceramides has been noted in both normal and affected skin of patients with atopic dermatitis [65,66]. The reduction in ceramides may result from increased sphingomyelin deacylace activity and reduced production of ceramides by keratinocytes from stratum basale to stratum granulosum [52,64,65]. Ceramides serve as important water-holding molecules in the extracellular space in the horny layer [6,67]. A deficiency in ceramides results in enhanced transepidermal water loss, dry skin, and increased permeability to environmental irritants and allergens [52,68]. In addition, keratinocyte-derived antimicrobial peptides known as cathelicidins and β-defensins are deficient in the skin of patients with atopic dermatitis [69]. These peptides help in the host defense against bacteria, viruses, and fungi.

Tight junctions function as the gate for passage of water and solutes through the paracellular pathway [54,70]. In addition, tight junctions regulate the localization of apical and basolateral membrane components and the lipid components found in stratum corneum [54,59]. Tight junctions are composed of a number of transmembrane proteins such as the claudin family, junctional adhesion molecule A, tricellulin, and occludin[54]. Claudins are 4-transmembrane-spanning proteins that determine the resistance and permeability of tight junctions and include more than 24 members [71]. It has been shown that in patients with atopic dermatitis, impairment of tight junctions may be mediated in part by reductions in claudin-1 and that claudin-1 (*CLDN1*) might be a novelatopic dermatitis susceptibility gene [54].

The loss of skin barrier function makes the stratum corneum susceptible to colonization by *Staphylococcus aureus* [72,73]. *S. aureus* is found on the skin in over 90% of patients with atopic dermatitis [54,74,75]. In contrast, only 5 to 30% of normal subjects harbor this organism on their skin [54,74,76]. Anterior nares of close contacts of patients with atopic dermatitis are reservoirs of *S. aureus* [77]. It has been shown that close contacts of patients with atopic dermatitis have the same strains of *S. aureus* based on molecular techniques [78,79]. The high prevalence of colonization by *S. aureus* may be related to increased adherence of *S. aureus* to inflamed skin, defective skin barrier function, decreased production of anti-microbial peptides, decreased innate antibacterial activities, reduced immune responses against *S. aureus*, and skin surface pH changes toward alkalinity [4,80,81]. Patients with atopic dermatitis may have exacerbations of the disease from overgrowth of *S. aureus* per se that can be independent of true secondary bacterial infection [81,82]. The severity of atopic dermatitis often correlates with the density of *S. aureus* colonization on skin lesions [54]. *S. aureus* expresses an array of adhesins known as microbial surface components recognizing adhesive matrix molecules that allow it to bind extracellular matrix proteins such as fibronectin and fibrinogen [24]. *S. aureus* exacerbates or maintains skin inflammation by secreting a group of exotoxins known to act as superantigens which stimulate T-cells, macrophages, eosinophils, and keratinocytes [1-3,83-85]. At least 80% of *S. aureus* isolated from patients with atopic dermatitis secrete superantigens [86]. Staphylococcal exotoxins exert proinflammatory effects through inhibition of apoptosis of eosinophils, increased surface antigen expression (CD11b, CD45, CD54, and CD69), and enhanced cytokine-activated oxidative burst, thereby triggering allergic inflammatory reactions [87]. Staphylococcal superantigens also have been shown to induce inflammation via the production of superantigen-specific IgE [54]. Toxin-specific IgE levels have been shown to correlate with skin disease severity [54,88]. In this regard, IgE antibodies to *S. aureus* exotoxins are found in approximately 60% of patients with moderate to severe atopic dermatitis [36]. Superantigens have also been shown to augment allergen-specific IgE synthesis [89] and to induce glucocorticoid resistance [90,91]. Binding of superantigen-specific IgE with respective superantigen leads to activation of basophils which may play a pivotal role in the initiation of IgE-mediated inflammation [54,92]. Colonization with *S. aureus* in atopic dermatitis lesions is often associated with worsening of clinical symptoms [77,86,93]. Re-colonization with *S. aureus* is frequent and may contribute to flares and severity of atopic dermatitis [77,94]. Recently, the cell wall lipoprotein lipoteichoic acid has been shown to be an important component of the ability of *S. aureus* to exacerbate atopic dermatitis lesions [95].Lipoprotein lipoteichoic acid acts as an agonist for toll-like receptor 2 as well as the platelet-activating factor receptor [95]. Travers et al isolated *S. aureus* from wash fluid obtained from lesions for quantitative bacterial culture in 79 of 89 children with clinically impetiginized lesions of atopic dermatitis [95]. The bacterial colony-forming unit (CFU) counts correlated with the Eczema Area and Severity Index (EASI) scores ($p = 0.04$). Lipoprotein lipoteichoic acid levels as high as 9.8 μg/ml were present in the wash fluid samples, and the amounts correlated with the lesional EASI scores ($p = 0.01$) and *S. aureus* CFU ($p < 0.001$) [95].

Malassezia (Pityrosporum orbiculare/ovale) has been identified as a trigger factor. Colonization with *Malassezia* is common in patients with atopic dermatitis and healthy individuals, with detection rates of 100% and 78%, respectively [96]. The head and neck areas are 7 to 19 times more likely to be colonized with *Malassezia* than the limb and trunk areas, respectively [97]. *Malassezia*-specific IgE antibodies have been found in 50 to 70% of adult patients with atopic dermatitis [59,98]. Patients with atopic dermatitis affecting the head and neck area are more likely to produce *Malassezia*-specific IgE antibodies [83]. It has been shown that internalization of *Malassezia*can cause maturation of dendritic cells and production of proinflammatory cytokines [83,99]. Some authors suggest that treatment with antifungal agents in postpubertal susceptible patients with refractory atopic dermatitis involving the head and neck may reduce the overall severity of atopic dermatitis [52,67].In a randomized, double-blind, controlled trial, however, the addition of antifungal agent does not seem to provide extra benefit to children with atopic dermatitis, and the beneficial effect of this medication seems to be restricted to a small subset of adult patients with dermatitis affecting the head and neck region [100].

The increase in prevalence of atopic dermatitis has been attributed to decreased exposure to microorganisms in early life, especially in developed countries [10,67,83,101]. Decreased rates of atopic dermatitis have been observed in individuals with greater exposure to infections, especially before one year of age [26,102]. Other authors suggest that exposure to specific microbes in the commensal gut microflora are more important than sporadic infection in the prevention of atopic dermatitis [103,104]. Watanabe et al have shown that patients with atopic dermatitis have lower counts of *Bifidobacterium* in their stools than healthy control subjects [104]. *Bifidobacterium* is a commensal bacterium that induces T-helper 1 responses [104]. Schmitt et al followed a cohort of 370 children not diagnosed as having atopic dermatitis during the first year of life [105]. For each individual child the authors identified all infections and prescriptions of antibiotics within the first year as well as incident atopic dermatitis within the second year of life. Stratified analysis indicated that early infections were only associated with a higher rate of atopic dermatitis when treated with broad-spectrum antibiotics such as cephalosporins or macrolides. The authors conclude that antibiotic treatment appears to modify the association between early infections and subsequent atopic dermatitis and there is no evidence that infections per se significantly alter the likelihood for subsequent atopic dermatitis.

A central neuroendocrine dysfunction may also have a role to play in the pathogenesis of atopic dermatitis. In the acute phase of atopic dermatitis, there is a reduction in the serum levels of both melatonin and β-endorphin [106]. Melatonin provides a homeostatic link between the brain and the immune system [106]. It has been shown that melatonin, via nuclear receptors, is responsible for most of its immune effects [106]. Melatonin has specific high affinity-binding sites on both T-helper 1 and T-helper 2 cells [106]. It has also been shown that serum levels of brain-derived neurotrophic factor and substance P correlate positively with disease activity and quality of life score in patients with atopic dermatitis [4,107]. Brain-derived neurotrophic factor is found in the nervous system and also produced, stored, and released by human circulating eosinophils [107]. Eosinophil apoptosis is inhibited bybrain-derived neurotrophic factor [108]. Substance P is a neuropeptide that works via a neuroimmunocutaneous mechanism.

Environmental factors such as food allergens, aeroallergens, heavy metals, contactants, stress, and mechanical stimulation may trigger or exacerbate atopic dermatitis in susceptible individuals [1-3,9,101]. Food allergy plays an important immunopathogenic role in 30 to 50% of young children with moderate to severe atopic dermatitis [49,80,102,109-111]. This is especially so if the atopic dermatitis is uncontrolled despite optimum management, particularly if associated with gut dysmotility or failure to thrive [15,16]. It has been shown that patients with atopic dermatitis have a facilitated absorption from IgE molecules present on epithelial cells of the bowel, followed by increased antigen transfer across the gut barrier [36]. Making an accurate diagnosis of food allergy can be difficult because other confounding factors influencing the subjective interpretation have to be excluded [112]. The delayed onset of symptoms (2 or more hours) after food challenge makes observation difficult, although up to 25% will present within 1 to 2 hours after ingestion of food allergen [112]. Moreover, results from a single challenge may be different from those with chronic exposure [112,113]. Burks et al evaluated 46 patients with atopic dermatitis for food hypersensitivity with double-blind placebo-controlled food challenges [114]. Sixty five food challenges were performed; 27 (42%) were interpreted as positive in 15 (33%) patients. Sampson et al studied 350 patients with severe atopic dermatitis for possible food hypersensitivity [113,115]. Food allergy was diagnosed by double-blind placebo-controlled food challenges. Cutaneous reactions developed in 75% of the positive challenges within minutes to 2 hours, but only 30% of the positive responses were isolated cutaneous symptoms alone. Most of the skin manifestations consisted of a marked pruritic, erythematous rash that developed in sites with a predilection for atopic dermatitis. According to the authors, a single ingestion of food allergen may not provoke an eczematous lesion, but chronic ingestion of a food allergen can result in the classic changes of atopic dermatitis [113]. Furthermore, children with food allergy may develop urticaria with ingestion of a food allergen when the atopic dermatitis is in remission, but the same food allergen can elicit eczematous eruptions when their disease is active [116]. Breuer et al performed 106 double-blind placebo-controlled food challenges to cow milk, egg, wheat, and soy on 64 children with atopic dermatitis [117]. Twenty-eight (57%) of the 49 positive reactions resulted in late eczematous reactions, either isolated or in combination with immediate reactions. Hill and Hosking evaluated 487 infants who had skin prick tests to cow milk, egg, and peanut and who had a family history of atopic dermatitis, asthma, fever or immediate food allergy in a parent or sibling [118]. One hundred and forty one (28.9%) of these infants had atopic dermatitis to the age of 12 months. These authors found that as the severity of atopic dermatitis increased so did the prevalence of IgE-mediated food allergy and the frequency of reported adverse food allergy reactions. The relative risk of an infant with atopic dermatitis having IgE-mediated food allergy is 5.9 for the most severely affected group. In a study of 95 children with atopic dermatitis, adverse reactions to food were found in 15.8% of cases [27]. The prevalence of IgE-mediated allergy was 8.4% [27]. The most frequently implicated foods include eggs, cow milk, tree nut, peanut, soy, wheat, seafood, citrus fruits, and chocolate [49,109,119].

Many patients with atopic dermatitis may not have overt symptoms of food allergy but are sensitized to common food items.Hon et al evaluated whether any association existed between atopic dermatitis severity, quality of life, total IgE, eosinophil counts, and the number of food items sensitized [120].Specific IgE levels of ten common food items were measured for a group of consecutive atopic dermatitis patients (n = 85) and correlated the findings with eczema severity.Twenty-four patients (28%) were negative for any of the ten common food items.The most commonly sensitized foods were shrimp (54%), egg white (43%), wheat (42%), and peanut (41%).Atopy to beef as a protein and atopy to orange as a fruit were least common among the food items studied.Patients with severe atopic dermatitis (objective SCORAD > 40) were more likely to be positive for at least one of the food items. The Spearman coefficients between the number of positive food-specific IgE and total SCORAD, objective SCORAD, area of atopic dermatitis involvement, Children's Dermatology Life Quality Index (CDLQI), total IgE levels, and eosinophil counts were 0.42 ($p < 0.001$), 0.45 ($p < 0.001$), 0.50 ($p < 0.001$), 0.17 ($p = 0.116$), 0.80 ($p < 0.001$), and 0.22 ($p = 0.043$), respectively. The number of common food items sensitized correlated with disease severity, extent, and total IgE levels.Approximately 30 to 40% of children lose their food hypersensitivity after 1 to 2 years of allergen avoidance and 80 to 85% outgrow their food allergies by 10 years of age [111,119]. Hypersensitivity to peanut, tree nut, and shellfish tends to be more persistent, with perhaps only 5 to 10% outgrow peanut allergy [119].

Aeroallergens such as house dust mites, animal dander, molds, and pollens may cause exacerbations of atopic dermatitis [36,121-123]. Intranasal or bronchial inhalation challenge with these aeroallergens can lead to worsening of the skin lesions in patients with atopic dermatitis [124,125]. Tupker et al subjected 20 patients with atopic dermatitis to bronchial provocations with house dust mite [125]. In nine of 20 patients, bronchial challenge induced unequivocal skin symptoms after 1.5 to 17 hours. Pruritic erythematous lesions on noninvolved sites together with exacerbations of existing lesions were seen in three patients. Three patients had an exacerbation only, and three other patients had new lesions only. As such, the respiratory route might be important in the induction and exacerbation of atopic dermatitis by aeroallergens [36]. In general, the degree of IgE sensitization is correlated with the severity of atopic dermatitis [124]. It has been shown that children exposed to environmental tobacco smoke are at a higher risk of developing atopic dermatitis [126-129].

Air and food pollution with heavy metals have been considered as possible culprits [130].Hon and colleagues evaluated if quality of life and severity of atopic dermatitis are associated with abnormal serum levels of six common heavy metals, namely, cadmium, lead, mercury, selenium, copper, and zinc [131].A total of 110 patients with atopic dermatitis and 41 patients with miscellaneous skin conditions referred to the pediatric dermatology clinic were recruited into the study.Serum or whole blood was taken for measurement of six heavy metals from these patients. Severity of atopic dermatitis measured by the SCORing of Atopic Dermatitis (SCORAD) system and the Nottingham Eczema Severity Score (NESS) system and quality of life measured by the Children's Dermatology Life Quality Index (CDLQ1) were recorded.Serum levels of the six heavy metals were generally within the upper limits of local reference ranges. In patients withatopic dermatitis, lead levels were generally within normal limits but their levels were positively correlated with poor quality of life (CDLQI: correlation (r) = 0.22 and p < 0.05), disease severity (objective SCORAD: r = 0.33 and p < 0.005; NESS: 0.20, p < 0.05), eosinophil count, and log-transformed IgE.Copper to zinc ratio also correlated with NESS and CDLQI and was generally higher in patients with atopic dermatitis than in those with nonatopic dermatitis skin diseases.These findings help reassure parents that levels of heavy metals generally do not exceed the normal reference ranges.However, lead levels have significant correlations with disease severity, quality of life, and atopy.

Decreased plasma zinc concentration has been described in some patients with atopic dermatitis [132,133]. In animal studies, mice fed a diet that was zinc deficient showed wider and more severe skin lesions than control ones [132]. However, there is little evidence for the role of zinc supplementation on atopic dermatitis in humans [133].

The frequency of contact sensitization in atopic dermatitis ranges from 41 to 64% [134-136]. Nickel, fragrance, and neomycin are among the most commonly implicated contactants [134]. Contact sensitization may provoke or aggravate atopic dermatitis.

Atopic dermatitis may result from emotional stress [1-3]. Patients with atopic dermatitis may respond to emotional stress with increased pruritus and scratching, which will aggravate the lesion of atopic dermatitis [1-3]. A higher stress-induced increase of cutaneous lymphocyte-associated antigen^{+} T-cells has been demonstrated in the circulation in patients with atopic dermatitis compared to healthy control [137]. This suggestsstress may result in an increased ability of T-lymphocytes to migrate to the skin [137]. Stress-induced immunomodulation may be mediated by neuropeptides [138]. Neuropeptides, especially substance P and calcitonin gene related peptide (CGRP) have chemotactic properties both to neutrophils and lymphocytes [139].

Mechanical stimulation may trigger or exacerbate atopic dermatitis [101]. In patients with atopic dermatitis, epidermal keratinocytes produce a unique profile of chemokines and cytokines following mechanical stimulation such as scratching. Interleukin-16, a Langerhans cell-derived cytokine for CD4- T-cells, monocyte chemotactic protein-4, and eotaxin are over-expressed in atopic skin

[140]. Occlusion may be detrimental in atopic dermatitis [140]. It has been shown that occlusion with polythene film up-regulates interleukin-1α, interleukin-1 receptor antagonist, andinterleukin-8 in patients withatopic dermatitis [140].

Chapter IV

Immunopathology

Clinically unaffected and affected skin of patients with atopic dermatitis shows mild epidermal hyperplasia and sparse perivascular infiltration of T-helper 2 cells in the dermis [2,18]. Acute skin lesions are characterized by intracellular and intercellular edema of the epidermis (spongiosis) – a hallmark of atopic dermatitis [2,141]. There is marked perivascular infiltration of T-helper 2 cells in the dermis. IgE–bearing Langerhans cells are seen in lesional, and, to a less extent, in nonlesional skin of patients with extrinsic atopic dermatitis [2]. Eosinophils are seen in the acute lesions but neutrophils, and mast cells are rarely present [2,141]. Chronic atopic lesions are characterized by a hyperplastic and hyperkeratotic epidermis with minimal spongiosis and increased inflammatory dendritic epidermal cells [2,18,141,142]. Cellular infiltrate in the dermis consists mainly of macrophages and eosinophils [18,67]. The number of mast cells is also increased.

Chapter V

Clincial Manifestations

Approximately 60% of children with atopic dermatitis manifest the disease by the first year of life and an additional 30% before the age of 5 years [1-3,143]. Intense pruritus and cutaneous reactivity are hallmarks of atopic dermatitis [1-3]. Pruritus increases the liability of the surrounding skin to react to light stimuli with itch – a phenomenon known as allokinesis [67]. Pruritus often leads to an "itch-scratch" cycle whereby pruritus is exacerbated by scratching which causes release of substance P from cutaneous proprioceptor nerves with resultant release of histamine from mast cells in the scratched area [67]. Recent studies have shown that histamine 4 receptor plays an important role in the pathophysiology of itch in atopic dermatitis [144,145]. Interleukin-31 and tryptase are also involved [144].

The clinical manifestations vary with age and may differ during the course of disease [2,3]. In infants, the eruption often affects the face and scalp (Figure 1), although the extensor surfaces of the extremities (Figure 2) and the trunk may also be affected [1-3,146]. The term "milk scurf" or "milk crust" refers to the occurrence of yellowish crusts on the scalp which resemble scaled milk [4]. The diaper area is usually spared [4,37]. Cheilitis is not uncommon [101]. The nose is often spared and is referred to as the "head light" sign [67]. In older children and adolescents, the neck and antecubital and popliteal fossae usually display the eruption (Figure 3) [1-3,37,101,146]. In a prospective, longitudinal birth cohort study of children born to mothers with a history of asthma, a total of 411 infants were enrolled and followed up for 3 years with scheduled visits every 6 months as well as visits for onset or acute exacerbations of skin symptoms [147]. Fifty five infants had incomplete follow-up and were excluded from the analyses.

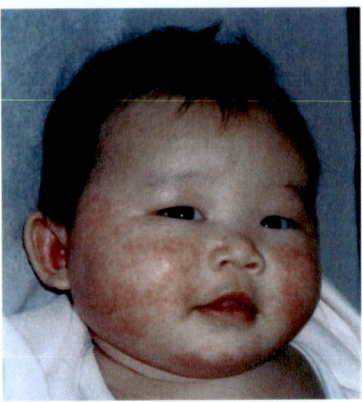

Figure 1. A 6 month-old infant with atopic dermatitis with extensive facial involvement.

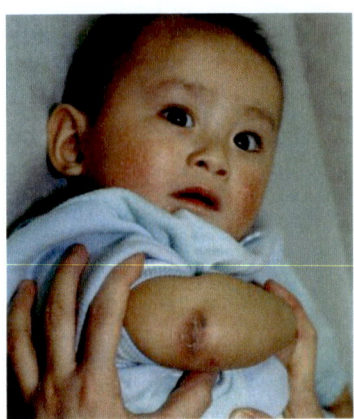

Figure 2. A 5-month-old infant with atopic dermatitis involving the face and right elbow.

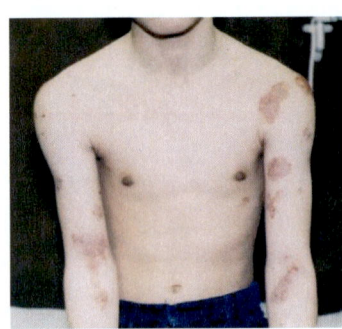

Figure 3. A 10-year-old child with atopic dermatitis involving the arms and antecubital fossae.

The cumulative incidence of atopic dermatitis was 44% (155/356) by the age of 3 years. Atopic dermatitis was found to begin at the scalp, ear, forehead, neck, and cheek and later spread to the extensor surfaces of the extremities, trunk, and finally to the flexor surfaces of the extremities [147]. In adults, eczematous involvement of the neck, hands, and flexures are typical findings and atopic dermatitis may present as dyshidrotic eruptions [37,101].

Lesions are classified as acute, subacute, or chronic and are usually symmetrical [148]. Acute lesions are intensely pruritic, erythematous papules, papulovesicles, or weeping lesions [148]. Subacute lesions are erythematous scaling papules or excoriated plaques [1-3]. Chronic lesions are characterized by prominent scaling, excoriations, and lichenification in classically affected body areas [1-3,37]. There is no central clearing [37]. Exacerbations and remissions are common and to be expected [37].

Xerosis results from reduced amount of ceramides in the skin with enhanced transepidermal water loss. Xerosis is seen in 67 to 98% of patients with atopic dermatitis [149]. Xerosis predisposes to the development of microfissures and cracks in the epithelium which favor the entry of allergens and microorganisms [18]. Other associated findings include Dennie Morgan lines (infraorbital folds), allergic shiners (periorbital darkening), palmoplantar hyperlinearity, pityriasis alba (Figure 4) [150], keratosis pilaris (Figure 5) [151], ichthyosis vulgaris [152], dermatographism, keratoconus, anterior subcapsular cataract, cheilitis, prurigo nodularis, and lichen simplex [153,154].

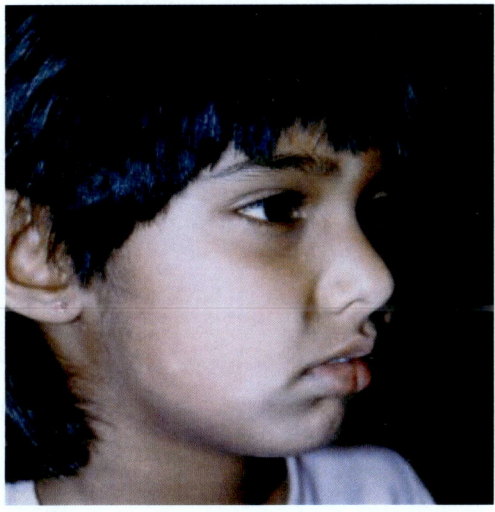

Figure 4. Hypopigmented lesions of pityriasis alba on the face.

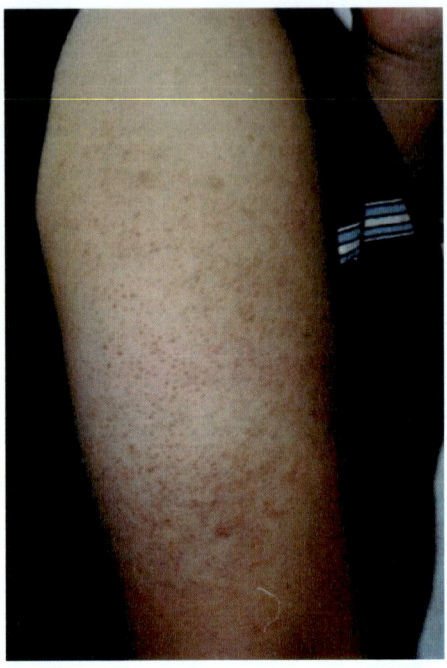

Figure 5. Lesions of keratosis pilaris presenting as minute, keratotic, follicular papules with variable perifollicular erythema.

In general, the skin manifestations of extrinsic atopic dermatitis and intrinsic atopic dermatitis are the same [9]. Patients with intrinsic atopic dermatitis tend to have a later age of onset and milder disease severity [9]. Dennie Morgan fold lines are more commonly found in patients with intrinsic atopic dermatitis [9]. On the other hand, features that are negatively associated withintrinsic atopic dermatitis include personal or family history of atopy, palmoplantar hyperlinearity, pityriasis alba, keratosis pilaris, and influence of emotional or environmental factors [9]. In intrinsic atopic dermatitis, no immediate skin reaction to environmental allergens or respiratory involvement can be observed [35].

Chapter VI

Diagnosis

The diagnosis of atopic dermatitis is predominantly clinical, based on a constellation of clinical features. Firm criteria to define atopic dermatitis were first established by Hanifin and Rajka (Table 1) [155]. While these criteria are useful for epidemiological and therapeutic studies, many of the features do not occur in children [154]. Also, the minor criteria have not been validated in a number of studies [154,156,157].

In 1994, the United Kingdom Working Party developed more straightforward criteria for the diagnosis of atopic dermatitis. According to the United Kingdom Working Party, atopic dermatitis is present if a pruritic skin condition is accompanied by three or more of the following: history of flexural dermatitis (or dermatitis on the cheeks in children younger than 10 years of age); personal history of asthma or hay fever (or atopic history in a first-degree relative in children younger than 4 years of age); generalized xerosis in the past year; visible flexural eczema (or eczema on the cheeks/forehead and on the extensor extremities in children younger than 4 years of age); and onset before age 2 years (for children older than 4 years) [158]. More recently, clinical criteria for the diagnosis of atopic dermatitis were developed by the American Academy of Dermatology Consensus Conference on Pediatric Atopic Dermatitis (Table 2) [159].

Table 1. Hanifin and Rajka criteria for the diagnosis of atopic dermatitis

Must have three or more basic features:
1. Pruritus
2. Typical morphology and distribution:
• flexural lichenification or linearity in adults;
• facial and extensor involvement in infants and children
3. Tendency toward chronic or chronically relapsing dermatitis
4. Personal or family history of atopy
Plus three or more of the following:
1. Xerosis
2. Ichthyosis/palmer hyperlinearity/keratosis pilaris
3. Immediate (type 1) skin test reactivity
4. Elevated serum IgE
5. Early age of onset
6. Tendency toward cutaneous infections/impaired cell-mediated immunity
7. Tendency toward nonspecific hand or foot dermatitis
8. Nipple eczema
9. Cheilitis
10. Recurrent conjunctivitis
11. Dennie-Morgan infraorbital fold
12. Keratoconus
13. Anterior subscapsular cataracts
14. Orbital darkening
15. Facial pallor/facial erythema
16. Pityriasis alba
17. Anterior neck folds
18. Itch when sweating
19. Intolerance to wool and lipid solvents
20. Perifollicular accentuation
21. Food intolerance
22. Course influenced by environmental/emotional factors
23. White dermographism/delayed blanch

Source: Adapted from Hanifin, JM; Rajka, G. Diagnostic features of atopic dermatitis. *Acta.Derm.Venereol.(Stockh).* 1980;92(Suppl):44-47 [155].

Table 2. Diagnostic criteria for the diagnosis of atopic dermatitis suggested by the AmericanAcademy of Dermatology

Essential features (must be present) • Pruritus • Eczema (with typical morphology for age and a chronic/relapsing history)
Important features (seen in most cases and add support to the diagnosis) • Early age at onset • Atopy (including personal/family history of such and IgE reactivity) • Xerosis
Associated features (help to suggest diagnosis but are nonspecific) • Atypical vascular response (i.e., facial pallor, white dermatographism) • Keratosis pilaris, hyperlinear palms, and/or ichthyosis • Ocular/periorbital changes • Perioral or periauricular lesions • Perifollicular accentuation, lichenification, and/or prurigo lesions

Source: Adapted from Eichenfield, LF; Hanifin, JM; Luger, TA; et al. Consensus conference on pediatric AD. *J. Am. Acad. Dermatol.* 2003;49:1088-1095 [159].

Chapter VII

Assessment of Severity and Psychosocial Impact

A number of scoring systems have been developed for the assessment of disease severity in children with atopic dermatitis. The SCORing of Atopic Dermatitis (SCORAD) system, Eczema Area and Severity Index (EASI) system, and the Nottingham Eczema Severity Score (NESS) system are user-friendly, relatively reliable, and in popular use [129,160]. These systems generate quantifiable data that are amenable to analysis [160]. The choice of which scale to use is a matter of personal preference. The SCORAD (score range, 0 to 103) measures the extent, intensity, pruritus, and sleep loss over the preceding three days [161]. It uses body diagram to record extent and area of involvement, and records the intensity of six signs, namely, erythema/darkening, edema/papulation, oozing/crust, excoriation, lichenification/prurigo, and dryness. It is a weighted index, with less weight on the extent (by multiplying a factor of 0.2) but more emphasis on the intensity (by multiplying a factor of 3.5) and symptomatology of pruritus and sleep loss (by multiplying a factor of 1) [161]. Hon et al have shown that subjective symptoms such as scratching and sleep disturbance do not correlate well with the disease extent or intensity [162]. Kunz et al suggest that a modified SCORAD index (without the pruritus and sleep-loss components) is more objective and accurate in assessing the severity of atopic dermatitis [163]. On the modified SCORAD grading scale, only objective items are used, namely, extent (20-point scale) and intensity (63-point scale). The total objective SCORAD has a 0 to 83-point scale [163]. A higher score indicates more severe disease.

Scratching lacks objectivity and is difficult to study. Limb-worn digital accelerometers have been shown to be a useful and practical way of assessing nocturnal scratching in the patient's own home [164-167]. It has been shown that nocturnal wrist activities measured with DigiTrac® wrist motion monitor (IM Systems, Baltimore, MD, USA) were closely correlated with the objective clinical scores and serum levels of chemokine markers [165]. Pruritus can also be assessed using instruments such as video recording [162,164].Sleep efficiency is also reduced and can be objectively demonstrated[168].

EASI incorporates body surface area involvement into the measurement. The index assigns proportionate values to four body regions, namely, head (10%), trunk (30%), upper limbs (20%), and lower limbs (40%) in patients 8 years and older, and is slightly modified for younger patients [169]. The six signs of atopic dermatitis, namely, erythema, edema/induration/papulation, excoriation, oozing/weeping/crusting, scaling, and lichenification are graded on a 4 point scale, ranging from absent (0) to severe (3). The EASI score ranges from 0 (clear) to 72 (very severe).

NESS measures the disease severity over a 12-month period. The disease severity is determined by evaluating three elements, namely, clinical course, disease intensity, and extent of examined atopic dermatitis [170]. Equal weighting is applied to the three parameters, each carries a score of 1 to 5. A final score is achieved by adding each score to produce a possible range of scores from 3 to 15, with higher scores indicating more severe disease [170]. The NESS is simple and quick to use and correlates well with the SCORAD scale [129,171].

Problems with interpersonal and intrapersonal variability are unavoidable when using subjective clinical scoring systems [162]. It would be useful for clinicians to have objective laboratory markers that correlate with the various clinical aspects of atopic dermatitis. Hon et al have demonstrated serum levels of macrophage-derived chemokine, thymus and activation-regulated chemokine, interleukin-18, and cutaneous T-cell attracting chemokine, and urinary levels of leukotriene E4 correlate well with the severity of atopic dermatitis [172-175]. Macrophage-derived chemokine and thymus and activation-regulated chemokine are not skin-specific and may be altered by other concurrent atopic disorders such as asthma and allergic rhinitis [176,177]. On the other hand, cutaneous T-cell attracting chemokine is a skin-specific chemokine and therefore more accurate in assessing the severity of atopic dermatitis, even in patients with coexisting atopy [173]. Cutaneous T-cell attracting chemokine functions by providing a skin-specific signal involved in localization of cutaneous lymphocyte-associated antigen (CLA) memory T-cells to skin and provides a potential target to regulate cutaneous T-cell trafficking [173,178].Using antibody array, more seromarkers are identified [177]. Correlations with disease severity are also demonstrated in other CC chemokines (such as CCL17, CCL18, CCL22), interleukins (such as IL-17 and IL-31) and neuropeptides (such as BDNF and substance P) [180,181].

A number of indices have been designed to measure the impact of the disease on the quality of life of affected children and the parents. Although some studies have shown a positive correlation between children's and parents' quality of life and disease severity on cross-sectional and over-time observation [182,183], there is not necessarily a direct relation between the severity of atopic dermatitis and its impact on quality of life [15]. The quality of life measurement provides additional information to the objective clinical scoring systems [183]. The Children's Dermatology Life Quality Index (CDLQ1) for patients 3 to 16 years of age is a self-administered validated simple tool to measure the impact of a skin condition on the quality of life over the past 7 days [183]. The index covers 16 areas including effects on emotions, social development, sleep disturbance, schooling, hobbies and treatment issues [184]. The score range is 0 to 30; a high score indicates diminished life quality [183]. The refined version of Childhood Atopic Dermatitis Scale (CADIS) consists of a five-scale framework, namely, family and social function scale, emotion scale, sleep scale, symptom scale, and activity limitations, and behavior scale [185]. It has 45 items and a score ranging from 0 to 180. The CADIS which assesses the impact of atopic dermatitis on both the child and the parent in the same measure, has been developed to assess outcome in clinical studies [186].

The Parents' Index of Quality of Life in Atopic Dermatitis (PIQoL-AD) is a quality of life instrument specific to parents of children with atopic dermatitis [187,188]. It has 28 items, covering a range of parental needs that can be influenced by a child with atopic dermatitis, such as need for rest and relaxation, need for self-respect, need for independence, and need for personal space and time [187]. This scale is particularly useful in those studies in which study participants are too young to provide information about their quality of life [186].

Suffice to say, the scoring systems for assessment of disease severity and psychosocial impact have often been used to assess outcomes in clinical trials [184,189,190]. The scoring systems are rarely used in clinical practice.

Chapter VIII

Differential Diagnosis

The differential diagnosis includes seborrheic dermatitis, psoriasis, acrodermatitis enteropathica, scabies, immunodeficiency disorders, nummular eczema, and contact dermatitis [154,191]. The lesion in seborrheic dermatitis is usually asymptomatic and consists of an accumulation of yellow greasy scale. In contrast, the lesion in atopic dermatitis is pruritic, the scale is dry, and excoriations are frequent. The diaper area may be involved in seborrheic dermatitis, whereas it is typically spared in atopic dermatitis [191].

In infancy and children, psoriasis often presents in the diaper area, elbows, knees, and scalp. The lesion is characterized by sharply demarcated erythematous plaques [192]. The thick silvery scale seen in adults is not common in infancy and early childhood. In atopic dermatitis, involvement of the diaper area is unusual and the lesion is always pruritic and poorly demarcated.

In acrodermatitis enteropathica, the skin eruption consists vesicobullous, eczematous, dry, scaly or psoriasiform lesions. In the face, it has a typical horseshoe appearance on the cheeks and around the chin [191]. In the perianal area, the dermatitis is erythematous and diffuse with a peripheral edge of scale [191]. Pruritus is not a feature of acrodermatitis enteropathica. Other associated features include chronic diarrhea, alopecia, stomatitis, glossitis, growth failure, irritability, recurrent skin infections, and superinfection with *Candida albicans*.

Both scabies and atopic dermatitis present with extremely pruritic lesions. In atopic dermatitis, the face is usually involved whereas in scabies, the face is usually spared. The lesions in scabies are polymorphic: papules, vesicles, pustules, urticaria, and nodules can occur all at the same time. Linear burrows are typical of scabietic lesions, and are not features of atopic dermatitis. In scabies, the lesions are often found in the web spaces of the hands and feet and other family members may be concurrently affected.

It is sometimes difficult to differentiate immunodeficiency disorders from atopic dermatitis in infancy. Pruritus is present in all of these disorders. The lack of localization, failure to thrive, recurrent infections, lymphadenopathy, and hepatosplenomegaly point to an immunodeficiency disorder [154,191].

Nummular eczema is characterized by coin-shaped eczematous plaques [3]. The condition is rare in the first year of life. The onset peaks between 15 and 25 years of age and again between 55 and 65 years of age [193]. The lesions are usually located on the extensor surfaces of the lower extremities and are often symmetrical. The knees, elbows, and scalp are often spared [193]. In contrast to atopic dermatitis, the unaffected skin in patients with nummular eczema is not xerotic [191].

Contact dermatitis is an inflammatory condition in the skin triggered by direct contact with an environmental agent. It may be irritant or allergic in nature. Both contact dermatitis and atopic dermatitis are extremely pruritic. An eczematous lesion conformed to the area of exposure gives clue to the diagnosis of contact dermatitis. It should be noted that patients with atopic dermatitis are more prone to develop contact dermatitis [134,136,154].

Chapter IX

Complications

Secondary bacterial infection, most commonly with *S. aureus*, is the main complication of atopic dermatitis [75,194]. The anterior nares are an important reservoir of *S. aureus* [73,195]. Recent studies have revealed an increasing prevalence of community-associated, methicillin-resistant *S. aureus* colonization among children with atopic dermatitis [76,196]. Suh et al conducted an observational cross-sectional study involving 54 patients with atopic dermatitis between 3 months and 17 years of age seen in the outpatient dermatology clinic of the Children's Hospital of Philadelphia [76]. Patients were excluded if they had symptoms of an acute illness or had current viral, fungal, or untreated bacterial skin infections. Swabs were taken from the lesional skin and sent for bacterial culture. Forty three (80%) patients were colonized with *S. aureus* and 7 of the 43 (16%) patients were colonized with methicillin-resistant*S. aureus*. Purulent oozing, honey-color crusting, folliculitis and pyoderma indicate secondary infection with *S. aureus* (Figure 6) [75]. Characteristically, patients with atopic dermatitis complicated by methicillin-resistant *S. aureus*infection present with facial/generalized erythema and a fishy odor [197]. The occurrence of methicillin-resistant *S. aureus*infection appears to be associated with disease chronicity and severity in patients with moderate tosevere atopic dermatitis [197].

Secondary bacterial infection may also be caused by group A β-hemolytic streptococcus (*Streptococcus pyogenes*) [54]. It has been shown that infection with group A β-hemolytic streptococcus is associated with severe atopic dermatitis [198]. Secondary bacterial infection caused by group A β-hemolytic streptococcus may result in poststreptococcal glomerulonephritis and posterior reversible encephalopathy syndrome [199].

Eczema herpeticum (Kaposi varicelliform eruption) caused by herpes simplex virus is a potentially dangerous complication [4,67]. Patients with eczema herpeticum may develop secondary bacterial infection, keratoconjunctivitis, viremia, meningitis, or encephalitis [54. Chickenpox can severely exacerbate atopic dermatitis and present as a generalized pruritic rash. Eczema vaccinatum, caused by variola virus, historically follows smallpox vaccination or exposure to individuals with or vaccinated with smallpox [200]. Children with atopic dermatitis are also prone to verruca vulgaris (warts), molluscum contagiosum, and superficial fungal infections [17,37,67,146].

Ocular complications of longstanding atopic dermatitis include eyelid dermatitis, chronic blepharitis, keratoconjunctivitis, vernal conjunctivitis, keratoconus, uveitis, and cataracts. Atopic dermatitis per se is a risk factor for the development of subcapsular cataracts, this is especially so for anterior subcapsular cataracts [201]. Atopic dermatitis may also result from the extensive use of topical or systemic corticosteroids [1-3,201,202].

Patients with atopic dermatitis are affected not only by the disease itself but also by the stigma associated with its visibility [5]. Postinflammatory hypopigmentation and/or hyperpigmentation may occur at sites of atopic dermatitis [37,203]. Hypopigmentation may also be a complication of topical corticosteroid therapy.

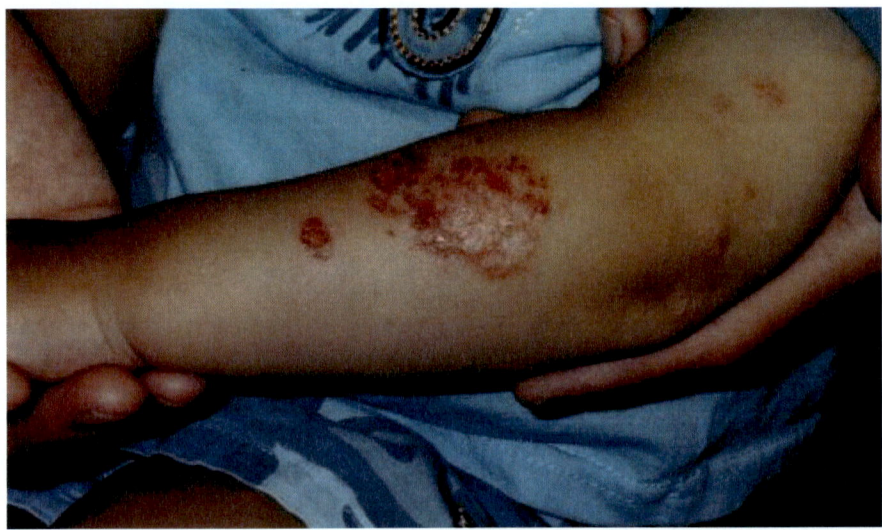

Figure 6. Lesions of atopic dermatitis on the left forearm secondarily infected with *Staphylococcus aureus*.

Atopic dermatitis can be quite uncomfortable and distressing to patients because of the associated pruritus and unsightly lesions [24]. Stress in turn can affect the atopic dermatitis. Children with atopic dermatitis may suffer from lack of sleep, loss of appetite, irritability, daytime tiredness, decreased school performance marked by an inability to focus, decreased participation in extra-curriculum activities, being teased by other children, emotional stress, low self-esteem, and psychological disturbance [5,204-208]. It has been hypothesized that circadian fluctuations in inflammatory mediators may account for increased sensation of pruritus at night and therefore affect sleep quality [207,208]. It is also possible that there is a common underlying mechanism of hyperarousability which may account for sensory hypersensitivity or reduced threshold for pruritus and disturbed sleep patterns among children with atopic dermatitis [209,210].

Quality of life is impaired in children with atopic dermatitis but the various aspects of quality of life may not be equally affected [179,211]. Hon et al reviewed CDLQI in 133 children (70 male and 63 female; age range 5-16 years) with atopic dermatitis [179]. Itch, sleep disturbance, treatment, and swimming/sports were the four aspects of quality of life issues that were most commonly affected, in 50%, 47%, 38% and 29% of patients, respectively. Problems with interpersonal issues (friendship, school/holidays, and teasing/bullying) occurred in only a minority of children ($\leq$ 10%). Girls had more problems with issues of clothes and shoes than did boys (odds ratio: 2.86; 95% confidence interval: 1.05 to 8.00; $p = 0.038$). Significant itch and sleep disturbance affected both genders similarly but were generally more common in children $\leq$ 10 years (itch, odds ratio: 2.31; 95% confidence interval: 1.04 to 5.14; $p = 0.039$; and sleep, odds ratio: 2.31; 95% confidence interval: 1.05 to 5.13; $p = 0.037$). The authors conclude that not all aspects of quality of life are affected equally in children with atopic dermatitis. The disease seems to affect personal domains of itch and sleep more than the interpersonal issues. Age and gender are relevant factors in quality of life with the issue of clothes/shoes being more troublesome for girls. Itch and sleep disturbance seem to be a problem mainly in younger children. Children's self-report of intensity of itch is negatively correlated with their self-report on quality of life and positively correlated with their depressed mood and catastrophic thinking [209,212]. It has been shown that patients with atopic dermatitis in childhood have a significant delayed social development in their course of life [5].

Atopic dermatitis may also adversely affect the relationship between the child and caregivers and may have an impact on the whole family. The disruption of school, family and social interactions can severely impair the quality of life and extends beyond the child [5,213-215]. Caring for a child with moderate to severe atopic dermatitis can place substantial demands on the caregivers [216]. Such demands include getting their children to take bath, providing them with optimal skin care, trying to comfort their children and prevent scratching, and ensuring the children to avoid allergens and irritants as well as to use proper medication for the treatment of atopic dermatitis [209]. Al Shobaili conducted a cross-sectional survey on the parents of 447 children with atopic dermatitis [217]. The parents were asked through a validated "Dermatitis Family Impact Questionnaire" about the impact of the disease on their life.For each questionnaire, a total score of 0 to 5 is considered as normal quality of life, 6 to 10 as low, 11 to 20 as moderate and > 20 as high alteration in quality of life. The severity of the disease was evaluated using the SCORAD index. The authors found that the mean score for quality of life in affected families was 13.9 (minimum 2, maximum 25). Based on the author's suggested classification, only 15(3.4%) parents had normal quality of life, 104(23.3%) were mildly affected, 297(66.4%) were moderately affected, while 31(6.9%) had severe alternation in their quality of life. Sleep, monthly expenditure, and food preparation were the activities showing the highest level of disturbance. Faught et el measured maternal stress utilizing the Parenting Stress Index-Long Form (PSI) in 33 mothers of children 5 years or less suffering from atopic dermatitis [216]. Mothers of children with atopic dermatitis exhibited significantly higher total stress scores (mean PSI: 259.6; 95% confidence interval: 244.9 to 274.3) as compared to mothers of normal children (mean PSI: 222.8; 95% confidence interval: 221.4 to 224.2) and children with other chronic disorders such as insulin-dependent diabetes mellitus (mean PSI: 218.1; 95% confidence interval: 204.7 to 231.6) and profound deafness (mean PSI: 221.7; 95% confidence interval: 206.4 to 237). Stress scores in the parental domain (138.2;95% confidence interval: 128.9 to 147.6) did not differ significantly from the scores of children with severe disabilities such as those requiring home enteral feeding (132.8;95% confidence interval: 125.0 to 140.6). Ratings of intensity of itch, whether made by parents for young children or older children for themselves, are significantly and inversely correlated with parents' quality of life [209]. Parents may experience guilt, frustration, resentment, exhaustion, and helplessness due to their child's condition [7,205]. Studies have shown that parents of children with moderate to severe atopic dermatitis often have sleep disruption and undue psychosocial distress [224,225]. There are also considerable economic costs associated with caring for children with atopic dermatitis [7,205]. Financial costs include purchase of medications, emollients, special foods and supplies; costs related to physician visits; and loss of income for having to take time off work to care for the child withatopic dermatitis [183,209,220,221]. The financial burden of atopic dermatitis for the society as a whole is quite considerable [222].

Chapter X

Diagnostic Testing

The diagnosis is usually based on a careful history and a thorough physical examination [36]. Laboratory tests are usually not required. Nevertheless, intrinsic atopic dermatitis can be differentiated from extrinsic atopic dermatitis by a normal total serum IgE and lack of specific IgE antibodies [35]. The need for diagnostic work-up has to be decided on an individual basis and should depend on the severity of the atopic dermatitis and the suspected factors involved [138,223].

Patients with intrinsic atopic dermatitis or extrinsic atopic dermatitis have peripheral hypereosinophilia [112]. However, hypereosinophilia in patients with atopic dermatitis is a nonspecific finding, as hypereosinophilia is also seen in patients with other conditions such as asthma, allergic rhinitis, parasitic infestation, Hodgkin disease, and Löffler syndrome. Although serum levels of macrophage-derived chemokine, thymus and activation-regulated chemokine, interleukin-18, and cutaneous T-cell attracting chemokine, and urinary levels of leukotriene E4 have been shown to correlate well with the severity of atopic dermatitis, currently their measurements are of academic interest only and have little use in clinical practice [224].

Approximately 70 to 80% of patients with atopic dermatitis have elevated serum IgE levels, which are often very high [6]. Patients with intrinsic atopic dermatitis usually have normal serum IgE levels [101]. Conversely, 15% of apparently normal individuals also have elevated IgE levels [225]. As such, routine measurement of serum IgE level might not be of use. On the other hand, IgE to specific food allergens is associated with earlier onset and more severe atopic dermatitis [49,226]. Radioallergosorbent tests can be used to screen for antigen-specific IgE in the patient's serum. Clinically, radioallergosorbent tests are used mainly in patients with severe atopic dermatitis and who have severe anaphylaxis [119]. Food-specific IgE has a high negative predictive value (approximately 75%), but the positive predictive value can be low (20 to 60%) [49]. Recently, diagnostic levels of specific IgEs to certain food have been determined and specific IgEs above these levels may have a positive predictive value of greater than 95% for food allergy [36,49]. It should be noted that patients with intrinsic atopic dermatitis do not demonstrate allergic-specific IgE [227,228]. Advantages of radioallergosorbent tests are convenience, safety, and the fact that the patient's serum can be tested for multiple different IgE molecules at one time [229]. Disadvantages include high cost, limited number of antigens available, delay in obtaining results, detection of circulating IgE rather than cell-bound IgE, interference with the test result by circulating IgG antibody, and the use of radiation with attendant precautions [110].

Allergy skin testing with food extracts is often used to screen patients with suspected IgE-mediated food allergies. The list of foods tested depends on the history and the age of the child [36]. A positive skin prick test merely implies the presence of food antigen-specific IgE antibodies and that the patient's symptoms may be related to the particular food allergen tested [110]. Overall, the positive predictive accuracy is around 40 to 50% [110,230,231]. A negative skin prick test, on the other hand, has an excellent negative predictive value (greater than 95%) and confirms the absence of an IgE-mediated reaction [110,230,232].

In the atopy patch test, aeroallergens or food allergens known to elicit IgE-mediated hypersensitivity reactions are applied to the back with large test chambers (12 mm) for 48 to 72 hours, with daily examination of the area to evaluate their ability to reproduce an eczematous lesion in the person being tested [134,233]. It is important to patch test only those areas that are free of atopic dermatitis, and recent application of topical therapy or phototherapy [225,233]. Before carrying out the atopy patch test, one should make sure that the patient is not on oral corticosteroid, oral tacrolimus, or oral cyclosporine and that the patient has received no antihistamine treatment for at least 72 hours [233]. Readings are performed according to the European Task Force on Atopic Dermatitis (ETFAD) guidelines [234]. After standardization, the atopy patch test may provide further diagnostic information in addition to the skin prick test and serum IgE values and it may be able to evaluate the actual relevance of IgE-mediated sensitizations for atopic dermatitis lesions [235]. An atopy patch test has a higher specificity (64 to 91%) than a skin prick test (50 to 85%) [14,230]. The atopy test is more sensitive than the skin prick test for diagnosing food allergy in young children with atopic dermatitis [235]. Of course, a combination of atopy patch test and skin prick test can enhance the accuracy in the diagnosis of specific food allergy in infants with atopic dermatitis [235]. Recently, the European Academy of Allergy and Clinical Immunology (EAACI) suggested the following indications for atopy patch test, namely, suspicion of food allergy or aeroallergen symptoms in absence of positive specific IgE and/or a positiveskin prick test; severe and/or persistent atopic dermatitis with unknown triggering factors; and multiple IgE sensitizations without proven clinical relevance in patients withatopic dermatitis [236].

The double-blind placebo-controlled food challenge has been considered the "gold standard" for the diagnosis of food allergies [49,110]. It has the advantage of objectivity. On the other hand, thedouble-blind placebo-controlled food challenge is time-consuming and has the potential for severe reactions [49]. As such, the test should only be performed by experienced health-care professionals who have access to emergency equipment [49].

Chapter XI

Management

Successful treatment requires a systemic multipronged approach that consists of avoidance of triggering factors, optimal skin care, pharmacotherapy during acute exacerbations, and education of patients/caregivers. Pharmacotherapy usually consists of topical application of corticosteroids or calcineurin inhibitors [237,238]. In a subgroup of children with severe atopic dermatitis, the disease is recalcitrant to conservative and topical therapy alone. These children may require systemic treatments such as oral antihistamines, antibiotics, leukotriene receptor antagonists, and systemic immunosuppressants [237,238].

Avoidance of Triggering Factors

Irritants, prolonged exposure to water, allergens, and emotional stress may lead to skin flares in children with atopic dermatitis [2,127]. Soaps, detergents, washing powders, fabric softeners, and perfumed products should be avoided as much as possible because of their potential to cause irritation and sensitization [81,121,127]. Soaps should have minimal defatting activity and a neutral pH. Nonsoap agents are least irritating and preferred. Chlorinated swimming pools are well tolerated by most children. After swimming, children should shower well and a gentle cleanser used to remove chlorine on their bodies.

Woolen or abrasive clothing should be avoided; children do best wearing cotton clothing [121,127]. The environment should be kept cool, if possible. Occlusive gloves, dressings, and fabrics should also be avoided [140].

The sensation of itch is often relieved by scratching which in turn may cause excoriation of the skin and possible secondary infection. Also, the first scratch initiates the second and this may become a vicious cycle [225]. As such, it is important to minimize scratching. To avoid injury to the skin from scratching, fingernails should be kept short, smooth, and clean. Light cotton mittens are occasionally necessary to control scratching at night.

Although total avoidance of environmental aeroallergens is impossible, measures can be taken to reduce exposure to these factors for patients in whom aeroallergens are suspected of playing a causative role [17]. Control of house dust mites may improve atopic dermatitis in patients who are allergic to house dust mites [18,239,240]. Schäfer et al examined the relationship between house dust mite exposure and atopic dermatitis and showed a positive linear correlation between them [239]. In the houses with the lowest house dust mite burden, 4.9% of the children had physician-diagnosed atopic dermatitis, compared with 13.9% of children in the houses with the highest house dust mite burden. Among recommended measures are use of allergen-impermeable covers for pillows and mattresses, washing of bedding in hot water, removal or frequent vacuuming of carpets and upholstered furniture, and elimination of plants and pets from the house. An indoor climate which supports the growth of mould, such as high humidity, should be avoided [239]. Household members should be discouraged from smoking [239].

Food allergy plays an immunopathogenic role in 30 to 50% of children with moderate to severe atopic dermatitis [1-3,102,109,113]. Most children with food allergy react to only one or two of the most common allergens such as egg, cow milk, nut, peanut, tree nuts (e.g., walnut, cashew), soy, fish, shellfish, and wheat [17,119]. In a well-designed prospective study of 113 patients with atopic dermatitis, marked improvement was noted in those who were maintained on an allergen elimination diet, compared with a similar group of patients who did not have food allergy or who did not adhere to the diet [241]. A Cochrane review of 9 randomized, placebo-controlled trials (n = 421) found little evidence to support the use of exclusion diets in unselected individuals with atopic dermatitis [242,243]. The current literature does not support routine dietary restriction for the majority of children with atopic dermatitis [133,244]. For children whose food allergy has been identified, elimination of the offending allergen from the diet seems prudent. Patients and caregivers must have a good knowledge of foods containing the allergen and must be taught to scrutinize the labels of all packaged food carefully [245,246]. Careful label reading is a cornerstone of food avoidance. Conversely, avoidance of common foods in children without documented food allergy might result in faddism, psychological dependence on an unsound diet, as well as vitamin deficiencies, malnutrition, and failure to thrive [36,246,247]. Children with atopic dermatitis-associated food allergy should be regularly re-evaluated for persistence of food allergy [36]. Approximately 30 to 40% of children lose their food hypersensitivity after 1 to 2 years of allergen avoidance and 80 to 85% outgrow their food allergies by 10 years of age [119]. The degree of compliance with allergen avoidance and with the responsible allergen may influence the outcome. Hypersensitivity to peanut, tree nut, fish, and shellfish may be long-lasting [36,246].

Presumably, delaying the introduction of solid foods may reduce the risk of development of atopic diseases by decreasing the dietary antigen load [133,246,248]. Studies on the proper timing of introduction of solid food into the infant's diet to reduce the incidence of atopic diseases are few and have yielded results that are confusing and at times conflicting [133,248]. The American Academy of Pediatrics recommends that feeding of solid foods be delayed until 4 to 6 months and whole cow's milk be delayed until 12 months [249].

Results regarding the protective effect of breastfeeding vary widely [250-252]. These might be related to methodologic differences and flaws in study designs (e.g., lack of control for compounding factors, failure to differentiate between exclusive breastfeeding from partial breastfeeding) [2,81]. The American Academy of Dermatology Guidelines Task Force reviewed the subject in 2004 and found no conclusive evidence that exclusive breastfeeding influences the development of atopic dermatitis [250]. There is, however, suggestive evidence that prolonged breastfeeding may delay the onset of atopic dermatitis [250]. In the same year, a group of experts of the Section of Pediatrics, the European Academy of Allergology and Clinical Immunology reviewed critically the existing literature and concluded that exclusive breastfeeding for at least 4 to 6 months in infants with atopic hereditary would result in a lower incidence of atopic dermatitis [251]. The present consensus is that in high risk infants, exclusive breastfeeding for the first six months of life is recommended which may delay or prevent the onset of atopic dermatitis [251,253]. Infants with elevated cord serum IgE or infants with at least one first-degree relative (parent or sibling) with atopy are at risk for the development of atopic dermatitis [109,254,255].

A recent systematic review by Yang et al (27 studies, n = 34,227) showed a summary odds ratio of 0.89 (95% confidence interval: 0.76 to 1.04) for the effect of exclusive breastfeeding on the development of atopic dermatitis [252]. Breastfeeding was associated with a marginal decreased risk of atopic dermatitis (odds ratio: 0.70; 95% confidence interval: 0.50 to 0.99) when analysis was restricted to the studies comparing breastfeeding with conventional formula feeding, but not with partial breastfeeding. When exclusive breastfed children with a family history of atopy and those without were compared, there was no significant difference in the risk of atopic dermatitis between the two groups. The authors concluded that there is no strong evidence of a protective effect of exclusive breastfeeding for at least three months againstatopic dermatitis, even in those with a positive family history. Further studies are required, with standardized methodology including controls for potential confounding factors and reverse causation, to substantiate or refute the protective effect of exclusive breastfeeding on the development of atopic dermatitis [244].

At present, the relationship between levels of transforming growth factor (TGF)-ß, fatty acids, and cytokines in breast milk and the risk of children developing atopic dermatitis is not yet clear [133,244,256].

When breastfeeding is not possible, a partially or extensively hydrolyzed formula is desirable [109,240,257-259]. To compare the incidence of atopic manifestations among infants fed 100% whey protein partially hydrolyzed formula and those fed regular cow's milk formula, Alexander and Cabana performed a meta-analysis on 18 studies representing 12 independent study populations [260]. The authors found that the risk of atopic outcomeswhich included atopic dermatitis was 44% lower in infants fed100% whey protein partially hydrolyzed formula than in those fed regular cow's milk formula (summary relative risk estimate = 0.56; 95% confidence interval: 0.4 to 0.77). In a sub-analysis of 4 high quality randomized studies (n = 749) that reported results specifically for atopic dermatitis, the incidence of atopic dermatitis was reduced by 55% (summary relative risk estimate = 0.45; 95% confidence interval: 0.3 to 0.7).

In the German Infant Nutrition Intervention (GINI) plus study comprising the GINI intervention study and the GINI non-intervention study, children with a familial predisposition for allergy whose parents agreed to participate in the prospective, double-blind intervention(n = 2,252) were randomized assigned at birth to one of the four formulas: partially hydrolyzed whey, extensively hydrolyzed whey, extensively hydrolyzed casein, or standard cow's milk formula [261,262]. Children with no family history of allergy (n = 2,507) or children with a positive family history of allergy whoseparents denied participation in the trial (n = 1,232)were allocated to the non-intervention group (n = 3,379). Follow-up data were taken from yearly self-administered questionnaires from 1 up to 6 years. The outcome was physician-diagnosed atopic dermatitis and its symptoms. The cumulative incidence of atopic dermatitis in predisposed children with or without nutrition intervention was compared with that of nonpredisposed children who did not receive intervention. Cox regression was used to adjust for confounding. The authors found that predisposed children without nutritional intervention had a 2.1

times higher risk for atopic dermatitis (95% confidence interval: 1.6 to 2.7) than children without a familial predisposition. The risk was smaller with nutritional intervention even leveling out to 1.3 (95% confidence interval: 0.9 to 1.9) in children fed extensively hydrolyzed casein formula. There is, however, no evidence that partially or extensively hydrolyzed formulas offer any advantage over breast milk [133]. Goat's milk, sheep's milk, or soy milk is not recommended in the prevention of atopic dermatitis in children predisposed to allergy [109,257,259].

Many authors are of the opinion thatextensively hydrolyzed formulas may be more effective than partially hydrolyzed formulas in the prevention of atopic dermatitis [247,261]. Recently, Iskedjian et al performed a meta-analysis on 6 randomized, controlled studies which compared the efficacy of a partially hydrolyzed whey-based infant formula versus those of extensively hydrolyzed whey- or casein-based infant formulas [263]. Themeta-analysis forthe partially hydrolyzed whey formula (n = 557) versusthe extensively hydrolyzed whey formula (n = 559) yielded a relative risk of 0.75 (95% confidence interval: 0.54 to 1.05) and 0.80 (95% confidence interval: 0.63 to 1.02) at 0 to 12 months and 0 to 36 months, respectively. Corresponding relative risks forthe partially hydrolyzed whey formula versusthe extensively hydrolyzed casein formula (n = 580) were 1.06 (95% confidence interval: 0.74 to 1.53) at 0 to 12 months and 1.13 (95% confidence interval: 0.87 to 1.47) at 0 to 36 months. The authors concluded that the efficacy of all three infant formulas in the prevention of atopic dermatitis is similar.

A Cochrane systematic review shows that allergen avoidance during pregnancy does not have a protective effect against developing atopic dermatitis and may lead to preterm births and reductions in birth weight [264]. The present consensus is that dietary intervention in utero is potentially harmful and is not indicated unless future studies prove otherwise [119,257,258,264]. In high risk infants, the avoidance of potent food allergens (e.g. egg, cow's milk) in the maternal diet during breastfeeding may have a preventive effect on the development of atopic dermatitis [239].

Emotional stress often exacerbates the skin lesions of atopic dermatitis. If avoidance is not possible, coping mechanisms should be tried [1-3].

Optimal Skin Care

Hydration of the skin helps to improve the dryness and the pruritus and to restore the disturbed skin's barrier function. As such,hydration of the skin is of paramount importance both in the prevention and management of atopic dermatitis [1-3,17,101]. Hydration of the skin can be achieved by daily baths in lukewarm (not hot) water for approximately 5 to 10 minutes, followed by patting the body dry with a towel [1-3,37]. Fragranced-free soap and cleansers are preferred [1-3]. The use of shampoo, bubble bath, and dishwater detergent to cleanse the body should be avoided [37]. Rubbing should also be avoided as such maneuver may precipitate the sensation of pruritus.

A moisturizer or emollient should be applied within 3 minutes to prevent evaporation of water and to keep the skin soft and flexible [154,159,265-267]. This "soak and seal" method helps to improve the integrity of the skin barrier and prevents the penetration by bacteria, irritants and allergens [13,268]. Bathing without moisturizer may compromise skin hydration. Ointments are most effective but messy; creams are often better tolerated. The type of moisturizer or emollient should be tailored to the individual skin conditions as well as the child's needs and preferences [15,30]. In areas rich with sebaceous glands such as the face, formulations should contain less oil than on other body areas [30]. Lotions, which have a high water and low oil content, can worsen xerosis via evaporation and should therefore be avoided. A dye-free, fragrance-free moisturizer should be used [81]. Frequent applications of moisturizers throughout the day help to maintain a high level of hydration in the stratum corneum [2,268]. Moisturizers containing urea, alpha-hydroxy acids, ceramides, or hyaluronic acis have been shown to improve the integrity of stratum corneum [13,53,269,270]. In this regard, urea should not be used in infants and toddlers because it often irritates the skin [127]. EpiCeram consists of a specific combination of ceramides, cholesterol and fatty acids (in the ratio of 3:1:1) that mimics those naturally found in the skin [271-273]. Recent studies have shown that EpiCeram has similar efficacy compared to a mid-potency topical corticosteroid but has a favorable safety profile [53,271,273].

Hon et al recruited 33 patients (mean age: 12 years; SD: 4 years) with atopic dermatitis to study the clinical and biophysiological effects of twice-daily application of apseudo-ceramidecontaining cream (Curel®, Kao, Japan)[274].Four weeks following the use of the pseudo-ceramide cream, the skin hydration,measured in arbitrary units with a corneometer, significantly improved(mean (SD) from 30 (15) to 38 (15), $p = 0.039$).There was no deterioration in transepidermal water loss (TEWL),eczema severity, or quality of life in these patients. The pseudo-ceramide cream improved the skin hydration (SH)but not the severity or quality of life over a 4-week usage [274].

Atopiclair, also known as MAS063DP or Zarzenda, a hydrolipidic cream, has been found effective in the treatment of mild to moderate atopic dermatitis in both children and adults [231,272]. The cream contains *Vitis vinifera* (grapevine) extract with antioxidant and antiprotease activity, glycyrrhetinic acid with antipruritic and anti-inflammatory properties, and hyaluronic acid which helps to moisturize the epidermis and restore barrier function [57,231,266,275]. Liberal amounts of moisturizers should be used which can be conveniently estimated based on body surface area instead of the less readily available tools for disease severity, degree of skin hydration, or skin integrity [276]. Moisturizers should always be used, even when the skin is clear of active lesions, recognizing that normal-appearing skin in patients with atopic dermatitis may not be immunologically normal [15,268]. Proper moisturizer therapy can reduce the frequency of flares and reduce the demand of topical corticosteroids or topical calcineurin inhibitors [53,57,132,266,277].

Topical Corticosteroids

Topical corticosteroids are the mainstay of therapy for atopic dermatitis, with the choice of potency depending on the severity, site, and extent of the outbreak [1-3,81,132]. Corticosteroids mediate their anti-inflammatory effects through binding to a cytoplasmic glucocorticoid receptor in the target cells and forming complexes that enter the nucleus of the cell [278]. Once inside the nucleus, the corticosteroid-receptor complex interacts with glucocorticoid-response elements and alters transcription of various proinflammatory genes, with resultant suppression of inflammatory cell lines and cytokines [279]. They also are effective in reducing the density of *S. aureus* on affected skin [13]. Topical corticosteroids are available in extremely high (class 1) to low (class 7) potencies [13]. In general, the least potent corticosteroid that can control the symptom should be used, and only low-potency agents should be applied to the facial skin, genitalia, and intertriginous areas. High-potency corticosteroids should only be used for up to three weeks for acute exacerbation of atopic dermatitis [18]. Topical corticosteroids should not be applied more than twice a day; frequent use does not improve efficacy and increase the risk of side effects [1-3,15]. Once daily application has been shown to be effective for topical fluticasone propionate and mometasone furoate [280,281]. In general, a gap of 30 to 60 minutes between the application of corticosteroid and moisturizer is desirable to ensure that corticosteroid is not diluted [282]. The medication should be applied gently as rapid rubbing may increase the itch sensation and result in scratching [282].

The risk of side effects depends on the potency of the corticosteroid, concomitant use of occlusion, the area being covered, skin integrity, and duration of treatment [1-3,57,203]. In general, non-fluorinated corticosteroids are less potent and show less adverse effects [101]. Compared with adults, children are at higher risk of both local and systemic effects. Local adverse effects particularly on delicate skin areas include skin atrophy, striae, depigmentation, telangiectasia, decreased subcutaneous adipose tissue, rosacea, perioral dermatitis, folliculitis, and steroid acne [1-3,17]. Percutaneous absorption of corticosteroids may lead to systemic side effects which include Cushing syndrome, hypothalamic-pituitary-adrenal suppression, cataracts, glaucoma, osteopenia/osteoporosis, and growth retardation [1-3,17,283]. Topical corticosteroids should be used with caution near the eyes to minimize the risk of cataracts and glaucoma. Suffice to say, systemic side effects are rare when topical corticosteroids are used properly [81,284]. Rebound flares may occur following discontinuation of therapy [101]. Tachyphylaxis may occur with prolonged treatment [15]. Should tachyphylaxis develop, a different topical corticosteroid of the same potency should be considered as an alternative to stepping up treatment [15]. Steroid fear or phobia among caregivers is common [101,247]. Suboptimal use of topical corticosteroids or poor compliance may account for at least some treatment failures [101].

Topical Calcineurin Inhibitors

The newly introduced tacrolimus ointment and pimecrolimus cream work by binding to a cytoplasmic immunophilin. The complex inhibits the activity of calcineurin to dephosphorylate the nuclear factor of activated T-cell (NF-AT), a transcription factor required to activate interleukin-2 gene transcription. Inhibition of interleukin-2 production blocks the activation of T-helper cells and T-regulatory cells, and the activation of natural killer cells and monocytes [209]. The immune responses that stimulate inflammation are therefore down-regulated. Both medications have favorable efficacy and safety profiles [285]. Percutaneous absorption has been shown to be low and there is no evidence of systemic toxicity. Topical immunomodulators significantly improve the quality of life of children and adults alike, as well as their family members [189,190,286]. Effectiveness does not decrease with time, and the rebound effect sometimes seen after withdrawal of a topical corticosteroid does not occur [287]. For patients with stabilized moderate to severe atopic dermatitis, long-term intermittent application of topical immunomodulators to normal-appearing but previously affected skin is significantly more effective than a vehicle control at maintaining disease stabilization [228,288,289]. Sequential applications of topical immunomodulators with tapering of topical corticosteroids may limit the long-term use and adverse effects of topical corticosteroids, while maintaining clinical control of atopic dermatitis and improving quality of life [290].

Topical immunomodulators do not decrease collagen synthesis or cause skin abnormalities or depigmentation [291,292] and can be used safely over the entire body, including the face and intertriginous areas [293]. Treatment with topical immunomodulators may even reverse the steroid-induced skin atrophy in patients with atopic dermatitis [14,230]. Treatment with either topical tacrolimus ointment or pimecrolimus cream is associated with reduced level of *S. aureus* levels in lesional skin of patients with atopic dermatitis [279]. Topical immunomodulators, but not corticosteroids, also suppress superantigen-driven immune proliferation [230,294]. In a subset of patients with clinical insensitivity to corticosteroid, there is a positive correlation between *S. aureus* colonization and disease severity [86]. Some of these patients may respond to treatment with an immunomodulator, particularly those patients with head and neck involvement [86]. The efficacy can be explained by the fact that either topical tacrolimus ointment or pimecrolimus cream acts through the glucocorticoid receptor [86]. The most common adverse effect of topical immunomodulators is a burning or stinging sensation or erythema during the first few days of application in approximately 10% of patients [295]. Less common adverse events include varicella zoster infections and vesicular rashes [13]. Treatment with topical calcineurin inhibitors does not affect the normal responses to routine childhood immunization [296,297].

Tacrolimus (FK506), a macrolide lactone produced by the *Streptomyces tsukubaensis* - a fungus found in the soil of Mount Tsukuba in Japan, has 10 to 100 times the potency of cyclosporine [298]. The ointment is the first topical immunomodulator formulated for use in children older than 2 years of age [298]. In addition to its inhibitory effect on cytokine production, tacrolimus inhibits the activation of T-cells, fibroblasts, Langerhans cells, mast cells, and keratinocytes that may result in decreased immunogenic response to antigens [279,299]. It has been shown that tacrolimus enhances the production of transforming growth factor-β, while hydrocortisone does not [300]. Tacrolimus is available in two-strength; the 1% ointment for individuals over the age of 16 and the 0.03% ointment for children over the age of 2 and for adults who do not tolerate the higher dose. The medication can be used twice a day for short or intermittent long-term treatment of moderate to severe atopic dermatitis [13].

Pimecrolimus (SDZ ASM 381), a derivative of the macrolactam ascomycin, is produced by *S. hygroscopicus var. ascomyceticus*. Pimecrolimus 1% cream has been approved by the Food and Drug Administration for short-term and intermittent long-term treatment of mild to moderate atopic dermatitis in individuals older than 2 years. Pimecrolimus selectively inhibits the release of cytokine release from activated T-cells and mast cells [30,279,301]. In contrast to tacrolimus, it does not affect cytokine release from monocytes, fibroblasts, Langerhans cells, and keratinocytes [30,301-303].

Iskedjian et al performed a meta-analysis on 15 articles reporting on 16 randomized controlled trials on tacrolimus (n = 9) and pimecrolimus (n = 7) involving a total of 5,301 patients, of whom 2,107 received tacrolimus and 1,225 received pimecrolimus, and 1,969 patients as controls [304]. Tacrolimus reduced EASI scores by 65.6% at 1 month and 73% at 3 months. In contrast, pimecrolimus reduced EASI scores by 61.5% at 1 month, 60.3% at 6 months, and 61.9% at 12 months. Tacrolimus success was 51.5% above placebo at 1 month and pimecrolimus was 45.9% above placebo at 1 month, 24.9% at 6 months, and 16.1% at 12 months. The authors concluded that success rate for tacrolimus and pimecrolimus were statistically similar. However, tacrolimus rates were consistently higher numerically than those for pimecrolimus, and tacrolimus was used in patients with more severe disease [304].

Ashcroft et al performed a meta-analysis on 25 randomized controlled trials that compared topical tacrolimus or pimecrolimus with another active treatment such as topical corticosteroids or vehicle in patients with atopic dermatitis and that reported efficacy outcomes or adverse events [305]. A total of 4,186 of 6,897 participants received tacrolimus or pimecrolimus. Both drugs were significantly more effective than a vehicle control. Tacrolimus 0.1% was as effective as potent topical corticosteroids at three weeks and more effective than combined treatment with hydrocortisone butyrate 0.1% plus hydrocortisone acetate 1% at 12 weeks. Tacrolimus 0.1% was also more effective than hydrocortisone acetate 1%. In comparison, tacrolimus 0.03% was more effective than hydrocortisone acetate 1% but less effective than hydrocortisone butyrate 0.1%. Direct comparisons of tacrolimus 0.03% and tacrolimus 0.1% consistently favored the 0.1% formulation, but efficacy differed significantly between the two strengths only after 12 weeks' treatment (rate ratio 0.80; 95% confidence interval 0.65 to 0.99). Pimecrolimus was far less effective than betamethasone valerate 0.1%. Pimecrolimus and tacrolimus caused significantly more skin burning than topical corticosteroids. The meta-analysis showed that tacrolimus was more effective that pimecrolimus. The difference was clinically but not statistically significant at the 0.05% level [305,306].

Paller et al randomized 1,065 patients to treatment in 3 multicenter, investigator-blinded, 6-week studies to compare the efficacy and safety of tacrolimus ointment and pimecrolimus cream in pediatric and adult patients with mild to very severe atopic dermatitis [308]. Based on the EASI, tacrolimus ointment was more effective than pimecrolimus cream at the end of the study in adults (54.1% vs. 34.9%, respectively; p <0.0001), in children with moderate/severe disease (67.2% vs. 56.4%, respectively; p = 0.04), in the combined analysis (52.8% vs. 39.1%, respectively; p <0.0001), and at week 1 in children with mild disease (39.2% vs. 31.2%, respectively; p = 0.04). Tacrolimus was also more effective than pimecrolimus based on the Investigator Global Atopic Dermatitis Assessment (IGADA), improvement in percentage of total body surface area affected, and improvement in itch scores ($p \leq 0.05$), with a faster onset of action. There was no significant difference in the incidence of adverse events, including application site reactions in the 2 studies involving 650 children. Adults treated with tacrolimus ointment experienced a greater number of local application site reactions on day 1; both groups reported a similar incidence of application site reactions thereafter. The authors concluded that tacrolimus ointment is more effective and has a faster action than pimecrolimus cream in children and adults with atopic dermatitis and their safety profile are similar.

Kempers et al randomized 141 patients (aged 2 to 17 years) to treatment with 1% pimecrolimus cream (n = 71) or 0.03% tacrolimus ointment (n = 70) twice daily for 6 weeks [307]. At day 4, local, application-site reactions were less common and of shorter duration with pimecrolimus than with tacrolimus. Incidence of erythema/irritation was 8% (6/71) with pimecrolimus compared with 19% (13/70) with tacrolimus (p = 0.039). Fewer patients receiving pimecrolimus (0%, 0/6) experienced erythema/irritation lasting > 30 minutes, compared with those receiving tacrolimus (85%, 11/13; p <0.001). Fewer patients reported itching with pimecrolimus (8%; 6/71) than with tacrolimus (20%; 14/70; p = 0.073). Incidence of warmth, stinging, and burning was similar in both groups; however, reactions lasting > 30 minutes were fewer with pimecrolimus (0%, 0/14) than with tacrolimus (67%, 8/12; p <0.001). The study was criticized for not adequately powered to detect a significant difference in efficacy response rates [237,308]. Although the authors concluded that efficacy was similar in both groups, after six weeks, there appeared to be a trend towards more children having almost or completely cleared atopic dermatitis when treated with tacrolimus (42% vs. 30%, p = 0.12) [237].

Yan et al performed a meta-analysis on eight randomized, controlled trials involving 1,781 patients aged 2 to 17 years to examine the efficacy of tacrolimus ointment and pimecrolimus cream in the treatment of pediatric patients with atopic dermatitis [309]. Primary outcome measures included investigators' global assessment or physician's global evaluation. Secondary outcome measures included EASI or modified EASI and adverse events. The authors found that tacrolimus ointment (0.03% and 1%) therapy resulted in the remission of atopic dermatitis; the effect was better than those of 1% pimecrolimus (p = 0.4) and 1% hydrocortisone (p <0.001) [309]. Recently, Chen et al performed a meta-analysis on 12 randomized, controlled trials involving 6,288 infants and children to examine the efficacy of tacrolimus ointment and pimecrolimus cream in the treatment of pediatric patients with atopic dermatitis [310]. The authors found that more patients using tacrolimus had a good response than in those using vehicle, 1% hydrocortisone, and 1% pimecrolimus. The corresponding odds ratios were 4.56 (95% confidence interval: 2.8 to 7.44),3.92 (95% confidence interval: 2.96 to 5.2),and 1.58 (95% confidence interval: 1.18 to 2.12), respectively. The effect difference between 0.03% tacrolimus and 0.1% tacrolimus ointments was not statistically significant (odds ratio: 0.9;95% confidence interval: 0.55 to 1.48). The authors conclude that tacrolimus ointments are superior to pimecrolimus cream.

In a recent, multicenter study of 347 patients with atopic dermatitis who had previously treated with corticosteroids, 171 patients were randomized to treatment with tacrolimus ointment and 176 patients to treatment with pimecrolimus cream for up to 6 weeks or until 1 week after the affected area (s) was completely cleared [311]. Based on improvements in EASI score at the end of the study,tacrolimus ointment was significantly more effective than pimecrolimus cream (p = 0.0002). Tacrolimus ointment was also significantly more effective than pimecrolimus cream at the end of study in all secondary end-points. Overall, the frequency of adverse events was comparable between the two treatment groups.

Recently, Doss et al performed a double-blind, non-inferiority study that compared tacrolimus 0.03% ointment and fluticasone 0.005% ointment in children with moderate to severe atopic dermatitis [312]. Four hundred seventy nine children aged 2 to 15 years with moderate to severe atopic dermatitis were randomized to tacrolimus ointment (n = 240) or fluticasone ointment (n = 239), twice daily until clearance or for a maximum of 3 weeks and, if the lesions remained, once daily for up to 3 weeks further. Primary end-point was week 3 response rate (improvement of ≥60% in modified EASI score and not withdrawn for lack of efficacy). Secondary end-points included pruritus and sleep quality, global assessment of clinical response, incidence of new flares and safety. The authors found that response rates were 86.3% with tacrolimus ointment and 91.5% with fluticasone. Moderate or better improvement on the physicians' global assessment occurred in 93.6% and 92.4% of patients in the tacrolimus ointment and fluticasone arms, respectively, while median pruritus scores improved by 84%

and 91.5%. Sleep quality improved by approximately 92% in both treatment arms. After day 21, new flare-up occurred in 5.5% and 11.3% of patients receiving tacrolimus ointment and fluticasone, respectively. The authors conclude that the efficacy of tacrolimus 0.03% ointment as second line treatment was not inferior to that of fluticasone 0.005% ointment, with similar benefits on global disease improvement and quality of sleep.

On February 15, 2005, the Pediatric Advisory Committee of the Food and Drug Administration recommended that a "black box warning" be placed on the topical calcineurin inhibitors, tacrolimus and pimecrolimus, because of the potential risk of cancer [313]. On March 10, 2005, the Food and Drug Administration issued an alert to health-care providers concerning a potential link between these topical calcineurin inhibitors and malignancy (skin cancer and lymphomas) [237,314]. The alert was used based on post-marketing case reports of malignancy among adults and children using these medications and studies in an animal study demonstrating an increased frequency of lymphoma when receiving oral pimecrolimus at a dose 26 to 30 times the maximum recommended human dose [16,315]. A Joint Task Force of the American College of Allergy, Asthma, and Immunology and the American Academy of Allergy, Asthma and Immunology reviewed the existing data and concluded that the current data do not support the use of "black box warning" on these medications [314]. In spite of this, the Food and Drug Administration issued a "black box warning" on the prescribing information for tacrolimus and pimecrolimus in January 2006 [315]. The warning includes the concern that the long-term safety has not yet been established and that although there is no causal relationship between topical calcineurin inhibitors and malignancy, there have been rare case reports in patients treated with these calcineurin inhibitors. The new labeling advises that these drugs are recommended as second-line treatments and that their use in children younger than 2 years of age is not recommended [316]. Clinical studies have indicated minimal systemic absorption of topical calcineurin inhibitors [17,57,266]. Existing data do not suggest the use of topical calcineurin inhibitors is associated with systemic immunosuppression, impacts delayed hypersensitivity response, or has an increased association with skin cancer [81,266,272,288,317,318]. Long-term post-marketing studies are ongoing to assure the safety of these products. Topical calcineurin inhibitors are particularly helpful in patients with atopic dermatitis whose clinical course is marked by frequent flares, disease persistence, and steroid tachyphylaxis [81]. They are particularly suitable for use on sensitive thin skin areas such as the face and genital areas [17,272].

Systemic Immunosuppressants

Systemic corticosteroids should be reserved for recalcitrant cases and used for the shortest time possible while awaiting response to other therapies [1-3]. International guidelines suggest that in the case of acute flare-ups, patients might benefit from a short course of systemic corticosteroids, but long-term use in children should be avoided [317]. Adverse effects of systemic corticosteroids include suppression of the hypothalamic-pituitary-adrenal axis, growth suppression, obesity, Cushing syndrome, hypertension, cataracts, glaucoma, osteopenia/osteoporosis, myopathy, aseptic necrosis of bone, striae, and increased risk of infections [238]. Rapid tapers may lead to rebound of atopic dermatitis [238].

Cyclosporine blocks T-cell activation and suppresses cytokine secretion [209]. The drug binds to T-cell intracellular immunophilin (cyclophilin) and the complex inhibits calcineurin [209,238]. Cyclosporine also inhibits the production of interferon-gamma (IFN-gamma). The medication is beneficial for severe atopic dermatitis unresponsive to topical corticosteroids [75,209]. It has been shown that cyclosporine significantly decreases symptoms scores, disease severity, pruritus, and sleep deprivation [209]. Atopic dermatitis might return after treatment ceases, although the severity is often less than before. A meta-analysis of 15 studies (n = 602) showed that the mean clinical improvement after 6 to 8 weeks of cyclosporine therapy was approximately 55% [319]. The disease relapsed in 50% of patients within 2 weeks and 80% of patients within 80% within 6 weeks after the medication was discontinued [319]. Adverse effects such as nausea, hypertension, gastrointestinal discomfort, hypertrichosis, tremor, paresthesia, hyperesthesia, arthralgia, myalgia, gingival hyperplasia, possible increased risk of malignancy, hepatic toxicity, and renal toxicity (arteriopathy and tubular interstitial disease) limit its usefulness and especially chronic use [101,238]. Due to concerns of development of skin cancer, phototherapy is not recommended during administration of systemic cyclosporine [101]. Cyclosporine is not effective when applied locally.

Various other systemic immunosuppressants such as azathioprine, mycophenolate mofetil, methotrexate, leflunomide, and recombinant interferon gamma have been used in a small number of patients with variable success [1-3,75,320]. These systemic agents all have significant adverse effects, requiring careful monitoring and restricting their clinical usefulness [13]. They should only be considered when cyclosporine is not suitable or does not produce a suitable response [209].

Antihistamines

Although pruritus in atopic dermatitis does not appear to be mediated by histamine release, oral antihistamines can provide symptomatic relief at bedtime because of their sedative properties. Antihistamines may be effective for intense pruritus refractory to moisturizers and conservative measures [1-3]. Breaking the itch-scratch cycle is essential for prolonged periods of atopic dermatitis control [238]. Of the H_1 antihistamines, hydroxyzine is more effective than diphenhydramine and cyproheptadine [321]. Side effects of H_1 antihistamines include somnolence, impaired cognitive function, hyperexcitability, and anticholinergic effects [238]. The second-generation antihistamines, such as terfenadine, loratadine, and astemizole, have few central nervous system effects and are nonsedating; they are also less efficacious in the treatment of pruritus. Nevertheless, second-generation antihistamines may benefit patients with allergic triggers and, with their chronic use, may decrease the rate of atopic disease [81]. Topical antihistamines should be avoided due to the risk of local allergic reactions and overall ineffectiveness [209,238].

Antibiotics

Antibiotic therapy is indicated for secondary bacterial infections that may exacerbate and complicate an acute flare [1-3,322]. Skin cultures and sensitivities should be considered before treatment as methicillin-resistant *S. aureus* may be an important pathogen in some patients [64,81]. Cloxacillin, clindamycin, first- or second-generation cephalosporins, or macrolides are most effective against *S. aureus*[1-3]. Maintenance systemic antibiotic therapy should be avoided because of methicillin-resistant organisms may develop [209]. Topical antibiotics, such as mupirocin, fusidic acid, and retapamulin are often useful on impetiginized lesions [1-3,323]. Clinical studies exploring the treatment of secondarily infected dermatitis reveal the efficacy of a 5-day course of topical retapamulin is comparable to a 10-day course of oral cephalexin [323-325]. Because topical use of antibiotics may induce bacterial resistance and contact allergy, topical antibiotics should be used with caution.

Some authors suggest intranasal application of topical antibiotic twice daily for 5 to 7 days to eradicate *S. aureus* colonization in the nares in healthy and hospitalized patients [73,230]. A recent Cochrane meta-analysis (26 trials, n =

1,229) failed to find any evidence that commonly used antistaphylococcal interventions are clinically helpful in people with atopic dermatitis that is not clinically infected [326].

Antiseptics

The main advantages of antiseptics over antibiotics are their much lower potential to reduce bacterial resistance and contact allergy [64]. Topical antiseptics should be considered in conjunction with systemic antibiotic for treatment of severely impetiginzed atopic dermatitis as well as for long-term adjunct therapy in patients with recurring superinfection due to *S. aureus* [64]. Topical antiseptics such as triclosan (2,4,4'-trichloro-2'-hydroxydiphenyl ether) and chlorhexidine have been used by some physicians to treat acute flares with clinical signs of bacterial impetiginization [101]. Diluted bleach baths are currently being evaluated for their role as adjuvant anti-infective treatment to break the cycle of repeated local skin infections in atopic dermatitis with heavily-colonized and/or superinfected skin [81]. A recent study showed that concurrent use of intermittent intranasal mupirocin treatment and dilute bleach baths might decrease the clinical severity of atopic dermatitis in patients with clinical signs of secondary bacterial infection [73]. However, it is not clear if the differences in favor of intranasal mupirocin treatment and dilute bleach baths are due to differences in baseline severity, differences in use of co-treatments, or a failure to undertake an intention-to-treat analysis [327]. Additional larger studies are necessary to confirm or refute this preliminary finding.

Triclosan-containing emollient appears safe and acceptable in the treatment of atopic dermatitis. Triclosan is a lypophilic chlorophenol biocide with a broad-spectrum antibacterial activity, highly active against*S. aureus*, *Klebsiella pneumoniae*, and *Proteus*species [64]. In a double-blind trial, Tan et al randomized 60 patients (aged 12 to 40 years) with mild to moderateatopic dermatitis to receive atriclosan-containing cream or vehicle [328]. All patients also received a low potency corticosteroid cream to use during the phase of study if necessary. At day 14, there was a significant decrease in SCORAD from baseline for the study cream compared with the vehicle ($p < 0.05$). At day 27, although there was an improved mean reduction in SCORAD from baseline, this was no longer significant ($p > 0.05$). Nevertheless, the amount of topicalcorticosteroid cream used by patients treated withthe triclosan-containing cream was significantly lessthan by patients treated with the vehicle. Further studies are necessary to confirm the corticosteroid-sparing effect of the triclosan-containing cream.

Chlorhexidine gluconate, a biguanide, is bactericidal to *S. aureus*[64]. It has been shown that the efficacy of chlorhexidine baths is similar to that of potassium permanganate baths in reducing severity ofatopic dermatitis and *S. aureus*colonization [329]. However, anaphylactic reactions tochlorhexidine have been reported which limit the use of chlorhexidine in patients with atopic dermatitis [330,331].

Silver or Silk Coated Textiles

Most of the silver or silk coated textiles are made from smooth materials minimizing irritation by clothing [75]. In addition, it has been shown that silver or silk coated textiles have antimicrobial properties and can reduce *S. aureus* colonization and toxin formation as well as severity of atopic dermatitis [332-336].Silver-coated textiles have been advocated as alternatives to antibiotics or antiseptics to reduce the staphylococcal load in patients with atopic dermatitis [322]. Gauger et al conducted a multicentre, double-blind, placebo-controlled trial on 68 consecutive outpatients with atopic dermatitis that was of moderate severity (SCORAD index $\geq$20) [333]. Patients were instructed to wear either silver-coated (verum, 35 patients plus 2 dropouts) or cotton garments (placebo, 22 patients plus 9 dropouts) directly on the skin for 2 weeks. Only basic skin care and ongoing therapy with topical corticosteroids or oral antihistamines were permitted. In the verum group, atopic dermatitis improved significantly after 1 week with further enhancement until the end of study ($p = 0.03$ and $p < 0.001$, respectively). Silver-coated textiles were comparable to cotton in wearing comfort and functionality. Pruritus and self-assigned skin condition improved significantly more than with placebo ($p < 0.001$ and $p = 0.003$, respectively). Juenger et al randomized 30 patients (average age, 25.5 years) with moderate to severe atopic dermatitis to receive silver textile (group 1, n = 10), silver-free textile (group 2, n = 10), and prednicarbate ointment (group 3, n = 10), from day 1 to day 14 (phase 1) [335]. In the second phase from day 15 to day 28, all patients wore the silver textile. In the third phase (follow-up period) from day 28 to day 56, no textiles were used. Prednicarbate ointment was allowed as emergency medication, but ointment consumption was measured. The initial SCORAD was 61.6 (interquartile range [IQR]: 26.6, min 30.6, max 99.9). At the end of phase 1, the SCORAD had improved significantly in the patients of group 1 (74.6 to 29.9; p = 0.005) and group 3 (57.8 to 24; p = 0.009). During phase 2, healing of atopic dermatitis continued in group 1 (SCORAD 29.9 to 18.1, p = 0.037), was observed in group 2 (SCORAD 48.2 to 24.1, p = 0.015), and remained at an improved level in group 3 (SCORAD 24 to 23.5). Median consumption of prednicarbate ointment (phase 1, phase 2, phase 3) was as follows: group 1: 135 g, 10 g, 45 g; group 2: 13 g, 0 g, 0 g; group 3: 145 g, 30 g, 90 g. Silver textiles reduced the severity of the pruritus (p = 0.031); silver-free textiles (not significant) and prednicarbate ointment (not significant) were less effective.

The use of silk fabrics coated with an antimicrobial substance has been shown to be effective in reducing the severity of atopic dermatitis in various clinical trials [337,338].Koller et al recruited 22 children (11 males, 11 females; age: mean 8.1 yr, range, 5 to 12 yr) with mild to moderate atopic dermatitis for a study period of 12 weeks to determine whether Dermasilk® (sericin-free silk treated with AEGIS™) was able to alleviate skin manifestations of atopic dermatitis [337]. AEGIS™ is a quaternary ammonium compound used on textiles demonstrating antibacterial and antifungal properties. All of them received three different tube-fabrics: Dermasilk®, sericin-free silk fabric without AEGIS™, and cotton, covering the cubital region. For the first 2 weeks of the study, parents were advised to dress one arm of their children with simple silk fabric and the other one with Dermasilk® fabric. After 2 weeks and throughout the rest of the study period, one arm had to be covered with cotton and the other with Dermasilk®. Evaluation of the local SCORAD score was carried out at the beginning of the study, after 2, 4, 8, and 12 weeks. A significant reduction of the local SCORAD index of the Dermasilk® covered arm was observed after 4, 8, and 12 weeks in comparison with the cotton-covered arm score [median (quartile 1 to quartile to 3)] 6.5 (5 to 8) versus 8 (7 to 9), p < 0.002; 6 (5.25 to 7.75) versus 8 (7 to 9), p < 0.0001; and 6 (5 to 6) versus 8 (7.25 to 10), p < 0.0001. Senti et al enrolled 15 children (6 males, 8 females) aged 0.6 to 9.2 years with moderate atopic dermatitis in a study to compare the efficacy of Dermasilk® and mometasone [338]. These children were given 2 sets of clothes. The left arms and legs of these clothes were made of Dermasilk® whereas the right arms and legs as well as the part covering the torso were made of cotton. The right arms and legs, which were covered by cotton, received 7 days of additional daily treatment of mometasone. The treatment efficacy was measured with a modified EASI and with an assessment by the patients/parents and by a physician. The authors showed that that was a significant reduction of atopic dermatitis after 7 days in all parameters, irrespective of the treatment. No significant difference between Dermasilk®-treated and corticosteroid-treated skin could be observed. At present, the use of silver-coated textiles and silk fabric in the treatment of atopic dermatitis is still experimental.

Coal Tar Preparations

The anti-inflammatory and antipruritic effects of coal tar preparations may help to reduce the amount of topical corticosteroid required in long-term maintenance therapy [101]. There are no randomized, placebo-controlled studies that have demonstrated their efficacy. Their tendency to cause stinging and irritation precludes their use for acute disease [18]. Disadvantages of tars are odor, dark staining color, and side effects such as folliculitis, photosensitization, and contact dermatitis [1-3,101]. The potential carcinogenic effects of tar have made this treatment lessfashionable. Tar preparation should not be used on acutely inflamed skin, since their use may result in further skin irritation.

Phototherapy

Broadband ultraviolet A and UVB, narrowband UVB, combined UVAB, and psoralen plus UVA (PUVA) have been shown to be effective in the treatment of refractory atopic dermatitis [25,75,339,340]. Presumably, UVA works by inhibition of Langerhans cells and eosinophils whereas UVB works by inhibition of Langerhans cells and keratinocytes [238]. Both UVA and UVB have been shown to induce T-cell apotosis [339]. UVB, in addition, suppresses the pro-inflammatory cytokines interleukin-2, interleukin-12 and interferon-γ [339]. UVB also stimulates keratinocytes to produce interleukin-10, which suppresses pro-inflammatory cytokines, and reduces natural killer-cell activity and lymphoproliferation [339]. Their use, however, is limited by the availability of lighting systems, cost, inconvenience, and adverse effects. Adverse effects include acute phototoxicity such as burns and pigmentation, potentially increased risk of skin carcinogenesis, and premature photoaging with prolonged treatment, particularly in patients with lighter skin types [238]. With exceptions, its use should be restricted to patients older than 11 years of age [1-2,75].Compliance to phototherapy needs further evaluation as patients might not come back regularly for treatment for prolonged period.

Wet Wrap Therapy

Wet wrap treatments are a useful adjunct for the short-term relief of pruritus in children with severe and/or refractory atopic dermatitis [81,341-343]. Therapy with wet wrap involves the use of an emollient under retention dressings (bandages or garments) [342,343]. Wet wrap acts as an occlusive barrier that promotes the penetration of topical medications into the skin and an effective mechanical barrier against scratching [18,81,341,344]. The evaporation of water from the skin surface results in vasoconstriction and cooling of the skin with relief of pruritus [154,343,344]. Wet wrap therapy also helps by debriding crusts from the skin surface and softening of the skin [18,341,344]. Such occlusive therapy is contraindicated if the lesion is infected [15]. Adverse effects of wet-wrap therapy include maceration of the skin with prolonged treatment and folliculitis if overused or used incorrectly [81,342]. Wet therapy may promote skin dryness if sufficient moisturizers are not part of the treatment regimen [81]. The National Patient Safety Agency (NPSA) has cautioned the potential fire hazard associated with paraffin-based skin products on clothing and dressings near an open flame [345].

Probiotics and Prebiotics

The use of probiotics and prebiotics in the treatment of atopic dermatitis is controversial. Probiotics are live microorganisms, which when administered in adequate amount, confer a health benefit on the host and enhance the growth of nonpathogenic 'good' microflora in the gastrointestinal tract. Presumably, probiotics mediate antiallergenic effects by stimulating production of T-helper 1-cytokines, transforming growth factor-β and gut IgA [346-348]. Examples of probiotics include certain *Lactobacillus* and *Bifidobacterium* strains. Prebiotics are nondigestible food ingredients that may help the host by selectively stimulating the growth/activity of nonpathogenic bacterial strains in the intestinal flora [349]. Ingestible oligosaccharides are the most common prebiotics used in infant foods [133]. Other examples of prebiotics include oligofructose, inulin, galacto-oligosaccharides, and fructo-oligosaccharides [133]. Several randomized controlled trials failed to show the beneficial effects of probiotics in the prevention or treatment of atopic dermatitis [350]. Other studies yielded different results [351-357]. In a randomized placebo-controlled trial on 250 pregnant women carrying infants at high risk of allergic disease, prenatal administration of

Lactobacillus rhamnosus strain GG (1.8×10^{10} cfu/day from 36 weeks until delivery) was not associated with reduced risk of atopic dermatitis [358]. In a double-blind, randomized placebo-controlled trial, perinatal administration of *Lactobacillus rhamnosus* strain GG has been shown to reduce the incidence of atopic dermatitis by 50% in children during the first two years of life [351]. A follow-up study showed that the preventive effect extended to the age of 4 years [351]. Viljanen et al randomized in a double-blinded manner 230 infants with suspected cow milk allergy to receive *L. rhamnosus* GG (n = 80), a mixture of 4 other probiotic strains (n = 76), or a placebo (n = 74), given twice daily with food for 4 weeks [356]. The authors found that *L. rhamnosus* GG was effective in alleviating atopic dermatitis in IgE-sensitized infants but not in non-IgE sensitized infants. In a double-blind placebo-controlled trial, Weston et al randomized 56 children aged 6 to 18 months with moderate to severe atopic dermatitis to receive *L. fementum* VRI-033 PCC (n = 28) or placebo (n = 28) twice daily for 8 weeks [357]. Fifty three children completed the study. The authors found that the reduction in the SCORAD index over time was significant in the probiotic group ($p = 0.03$) but not in the placebo group. In a double-blind, randomized, placebo trial, a mixture of probiotic bacteria (*Bifidobacterium bifidum*, *Bifidobacterium lactis*, *Lactococcus lactis*) was prenatally administered to mothers with a positive family history of allergic disease and to their offspring for the first 12 months of life [359]. Parental-reported atopic dermatitis during the first 3 months of life was significantly lower in the intervention group compared with placebo, 6/50 versus 15/52 ($p = 0.035$). After 3 months, the incidence of atopic dermatitis was similar in both groups. Cumulative incidence of parental-reported atopic dermatitis at 1 and 2 years was 23/50 (intervention) versus 31/48 (placebo) and 27 (intervention) versus 34 (placebo), respectively. The authors concluded that such combination of probiotic bacteria had a preventive effect on the incidence of atopic dermatitis in high-risk children; the preventive effect seemed to be sustained during the first two years of life. In a double-blind study, Passeron et al randomized 48 children to receive either *L. rhamnosus* Lcr 35 plus a prebiotic preparation (n = 28) or an identically appearing prebiotic preparation alone three times a day for 3 months [360]. In the symbiotic group, the mean total SCORAD score was 39.1 before treatment versus 20.7 after 3 months of treatment ($p < 0.0001$). In the prebiotic group, the mean SCORAD score was 39.3 before the treatment versus 24.0 after 3 months of treatment ($p < 0.0001$). The authors concluded that both synbiotics and prebiotics used alone were effective in the treatment of atopic dermatitis. On the other hand, in a double-blind, placebo-controlled trial, 253 infants with a family history of allergy were randomized to receive at least 60 ml of commercially available cow's milk formula with (n = 127) or without (n = 126) probiotic supplementation (*Bifidobacterium longum* [BL999] 1 x 10^7 colony forming unit/g and *L. rhamnosus* 2 x 10^7 colony forming unit/g) daily for the first 6 months [355]. At the 12-month visit, there were 124 families in the probiotic arm and 121 families in the placebo arm. The authors found that the incidence of atopic dermatitis in the probiotic group (22%) was similar to that in the placebo group (25%) (p = 0.53).

In a double-blind, placebo-controlled multi-center trial, 90 infants with atopic dermatitis (SCORAD score ≥ 15), aged < 7 months and exclusively formula fed, were randomized to receive either an extensively hydrolyzed formula with *Bifidobacterium breve* M-16V and a galacto-/fructo-oligosaccharide mixture (Immunofortis®), or the same formula without synbiotics for 12 weeks [361]. There was no difference in SCORAD score improvement between the symbiotic and the placebo group.

In a Cochrane's meta-analysis on 12 randomized placebo-controlled trials (n = 781) which evaluated probiotics as treatment for atopic dermatitis, there was no significant difference in participant or parent-rated symptoms scores in favor of probiotic treatment (5 trials, n = 313) [362]. Symptom severity on a scale from 0 to 20 was 0.9 points lower after probiotic treatment than after placebo (95% confidence interval: -1.04 to 2.84; p = 0.36). There was no significant difference in participant or parent-rated overall atopic dermatitis severity in favor of probiotic treatment (3 trials, n = 150). There was also no significant difference in investigator-rated atopic dermatitis severity between probiotic and placebo treatment (7 trials, n =588). On a scale from 0 to 102, investigator-rated atopic dermatitis severity was 2.46 points lower after probiotic treatment than after placebo treatment (95% confidence interval: -2.53 to 7.45; p = 0.33). Significant heterogeneity was noted between the results of individual studies, which may be explained by the use of different probiotic strains. The above evidence suggests that probiotics are not effective treatment for atopic dermatitis. Lee et al performed a meta-analysis on 10 randomized, double-blind, placebo-controlled trials [363]. Data from 6 prevention studies (n = 1581) and 4 treatment studies (n = 299) were pooled by using fixed-effects and random-effects models of relative risk ratios and of weighted mean difference, respectively. Prevention corresponded with summary effect sizes of 0.69 (95% confidence interval: 0.57 to 0.83) and 0.66 (95% confidence interval: 0.49 to 0.89), respectively, supporting the potential of probiotics in the prevention of pediatric atopic dermatitis, which decreased further to 0.61 after exclusion of one trial of probiotics given only postnatally. The clinical significance of the treatment trial findings of intergroup SCORAD score reduction by -6.64 points (95% confidence interval: -9.78 to -3.49) and -8.56 (95% confidence interval: -18.39 to 1.28) and intergroup change of -1.06 (95% confidence interval: -3.86 to 1.73) and -1.37 (95% confidence interval: -4.81 to 2.07) is questionable. In short, there are conflicting results regarding the effects of probiotics or prebiotics in the prevention or treatment of atopic dermatitis [364]. This may be due to different study designs in terms of selection criteria of patients, dosage of probiotics or probiotics, duration of treatment, length of follow-up, and time slot of administration [364]. At present, there is not enough evidence to support the use of probiotics or prebiotics for the prevention or treatment of atopic dermatitis [364-366].

Leukotriene Receptor Antagonists

Leukotriene receptor antagonists (montelukast, zafirlukast, and pranlukast) block the effects of cysteinyl leukotrienes by competitive binding to the cysteinyl leukotriene 1 receptor [209]. Cysteinyl leukotrienes are potent proinflammatory mediators and may have a role to play in the pathogenesis of atopic dermatitis [367]. Leukotriene receptor antagonists are usually well tolerated. Adverse effects include headaches, sore throat, and transient elevation of alanine aminotransferase. Preliminary studies have shown that oral montelukast has a corticosteroid-sparing effect and may be of use as an adjunctive treatment for atopic dermatitis [367-373]. More and larger randomized controlled trials are necessary to substantiate these preliminary findings.

Allergen-Specific Immunotherapy/Hyposensitization

Currently, allergen-specific immunotherapy is not an established mode of instrument for the treatment of atopic dermatitis [138,316]. Some investigators found a significant improvement of skin symptoms with allergen-specific immunotherapy [374-377]. In a multi-center, double-blind, controlled trial, Werfel et al randomized 89 patients with a chronic course of atopic dermatitis, SCORAD ≥ 40 and allergic sensitization to house dust mites (CAP-FEIA ≥3), to receive subcutaneous specific immunotherapy with a house dust mite preparation (*Dermatophagoides pteronyssinus/D. farinae*) at maintenance doses of 20, 2,000, and 20,000 SQ-U, respectively, in weekly intervals for one year [377]. Fifty one individuals completed the study. The SCORAD declined in the three dose groups in a dose-dependent manner (p = 0.0368, Jonckheere-Terpstra test) and was significantly lower in the two high-dose groups (2,000, 20,000 SQ-U) compared with the low-dose group (20 SQ-U) ($p = 0.0379$, U-test) after one year of specific immunotherapy. The use of topical corticosteroids was significantly reduced with higher doses ($p = 0.0007$, Mantel-Haenszel chi-square test). In a open-label study involving 25 atopic dermatitis patients (14 males, 11 females; mean age: 31.04 years, range, 5 to 65 years) with IgE-mediated sensitization against house dust mites, subcutaneous allergic-specific immunotherapy with an house dust mite extract led to a significant improvement of atopic dermatitis mirrored by a reduction of SCORAD as well as serological and immunological changes [374]. In another open non-controlled trial involving 86 patients (33 males, 53 females; mean age: 26 years, range, 3 to 60 years) with mild to moderate atopic dermatitis and IgE-mediated sensitization against house dust mites, sublingual allergic-specific immunotherapy with house dust mite extracts resulted in reduction of the SCORAD after one year of treatment [378]. The baseline SCORAD was 43.3 ± 13.7 and the SCORAD after one year of treatment was 23.7 ± 13.3 ($p = 0.0001$; unpaired t-test versus baseline). Pajno et al conducted a randomized, double-blind, placebo-controlled trial to assess the effect of sublingual immunotherapy in 56 children (5 to 16 years of age) with atopic dermatitis (SCORAD >7) and sensitization to dust mite alone, without food allergy or chronic asthma [376]. Sublingual immunotherapy ($n = 28$) or placebo ($n = 28$) was given for 18 months in addition to standard therapy. Forty eight children completed the study, with 2 dropouts in the treatment group and 6 in the placebo group. The difference from baseline in the SCORAD was significant ($p = 0.025$) between the 2 groups starting from the ninth month. Similarly, there was a significant reduction in the use of medications only in the treatment group. A trend toward significance was seen for the visual analog score only in the treatment group versus baseline ($p = 0.07$). A significant difference in the considered parameters was found only in patients with a mild to moderate disease, whereas severe patients had only a marginal benefit. Other investigators could not confirm their observations [379,380]. It is hoped that future well-designed, large-scale, randomized, placebo-controlled studies will provide more information in this area.

Complementary/Alternative Therapies

The use of complementary and alternative medicine is popular, in spite of lack of strong clinical evidence of efficacy. Based on the 2007 National Health Interviews of 23,393 adults older than 18 years and 9,417 children younger than

17 years, approximately 38% of adults and 12% of children in the United States used some form of complementary and alternative medicine [365]. In the pediatric age group, the use of complementary and alternative medicine in the treatment of atopic dermatitis is often based on recommendation from others (47%), fear of side effects of steroids (26.4%), and dissatisfaction with conventional treatment (17.6%) [381].

Traditional Chinese herbal medicine has been studied in controlled trials in the treatment of atopic dermatitis with variable success [382-384]. Unfortunately, some of the traditional Chinese medicine contain corticosteroids which produce clinical improvements and adverse effects caused by conventional corticosteroids such as cataract formation [385-387]. Some are less palatable. Some herbal preparations from China have been found to be contaminated with heavy metals such as mercury and arsenic and may have the potential risk of agranulocytosis, hepatic toxicity, renal toxicity, and cardiomyopathy [384,388-390]. Recently, Hon et al randomized 85 patients (aged 5-21 years) with longstanding moderate to severe atopic dermatitis to receive a 12-week treatment with twice daily dosing of three capsules containing five herbs (n = 42) which include *Flos lonicerae (Jinyinhua), Herba menthae (Bohe), Cortex moutan (Danpi), Rhizoma atractylodis (Cangzhu) and Cortex phellodendri (Huangbai)*, or placebo (n=43) [383]. The CDLQI in traditional Chinese herbal medicine treated patients were significant improved compared with patients receiving placebo at end of the 3-month treatment and 4 weeks after stopping therapy (p = 0.008 and 0.059, respectively). Adverse effects were relatively uncommon and were generally mild and self-limiting. A syrup form of the same concoction was tried on 22 children 4 to 7 years of age by the same authors [391].Clinical parameters and laboratory markers were measured before, at 2 weeks, 7 weeks, 12 weeks of treatment, and 4 weeks after completion of treatment.Disease severity was evaluated by the SCORAD index and quality of life by the CDLQI.Blood was obtained for complete blood count, total IgE, eosinophil count, and biochemical studies prior to and after three months of traditional Chinese herbal medicine usage.There were significant improvements in the objective SCORAD,pruritus and CDLQI scores 4 weeks after completion of the study. There was no change in sleep score or amount of topical steroid consumption.No biochemical evidence of any adverse drug reaction was observed during the study period.The traditional Chinese herbal medicine was generally palatable and well tolerated by children in the study.Adverse effects were generally mild but two patients with rash withdrew during the study. The authors suggest that further evaluations on the palatability and dosage studies of the concoction should be performed in young children. In a separate study, Hon et al showed that corticosteroids were not present in the 5 herbs used in the study [392].

Rosmarinic acid (α-o-caffeoyl-3, 4-dihydroxyphenyl lactic acid), a naturally occurring hydroxylated compound, is known to have anti-inflammatory and immunomodulatory activities [393]. A double-blind, vehicle-controlled, randomized trial was performed to evaluate the clinical effects of a cream containing 0.3% rosmarinic acid on atopic dermatitis patients over a 8-week period [393]. Rosmarinic acid (03%) cream was topically applied to the elbow flexures of 21 patients (14 females and 7 males, aged 5 to 28 years) twice a day. Cream without 0.3% rosmarinic acid was applied to the elbow flexures of control subjects twice a day. The mean SCORAD index decreased from 7.37 ± 0.32 before treatment to 3.27 ± 0.21 after treatment with rosamarinic acid-containing cream for 8 weeks ($p < 0.05$). However, in the control group, no significant change of SCORAD score was observed. Transepidermal water loss of the antecubital fossa was significantly reduced at 8 weeks compared to before treatment ($p < 0.05$). Further studies are warranted to determine whether rosmarinic acid can be used as an alternate or adjuvant agent for the treatment of atopic dermatitis.

Dietary essential fatty acid (in particular, omega-3 fatty acids and omega-6 fatty acids) supplementation has been studied for the prevention and treatment of atopic dermatitis. It has been postulated that atopic patients may have a deficiency of γ-linolenic acid, a precursor of prostaglandin E_1 and an important component of T-lymphocyte function [365]. Consequently, production of prostaglandin E_1 is diminished in patients with atopic dermatitis and the proinflammatory prostaglandin E_2 and prostaglandin F_2 predominate [133,394]. A recent systematic review and meta-analysis examined supplementation with omega-3 fatty acids (3 studies, n = 664) and omega-6 fatty acids (2 studies, n = 259) as a prophylactic therapy for patients at high risk of atopic dermatitis [395]. The pooled data for risk of developing atopic dermatitis following omega-3 fatty acid supplementation showed a non-significant increased risk in those who received the intervention compared to those who received placebo (relative risk: 1.10; 95% confidence interval: 0.78 to 1.54). The pooled relative risk for development of atopic dermatitis in those who received omega-6 fatty acid supplementation compared to those who received placebo was 0.80 (95% confidence interval: 0.56 to 1.16) indicating that omega-6 fatty acid supplementation had a non-significant protective effect. Hoppu et al collected food records and breast milk samples from 34 mothers with atopic dermatitis at the infants' age of one month [396]. Their infants were clinically examined for atopic dermatitis at one, three, six, and 12 months. Thirteen of 34 (38%) infants were diagnosed to have atopic dermatitis during the first year of life. Infants developing atopic dermatitis had consumed breast milk with a higher ratio of saturated to polyunsaturated fatty acids and less omega-3 fatty acids compared to infants not developing atopic dermatitis. Specifically, breast milk consumed by infants with atopic dermatitis contained more stearic acid, 8.9% of total fatty acids (95% confidence interval: 7.9 to 10.0) in comparison to those without atopic dermatitis, 7.1% of total fatty acids (95% confidence interval: 6.6 to 7.7). The authors conclude that breast milk rich in saturated fatty acids and low in omega-3 fatty acids may be a risk factor for atopic dermatitis in the infant. Unfortunately, maternal oral supplementation with omega-3 fatty acids and omega-6 fatty acids does not reduce the incidence of atopic dermatitis in their infants [133,397-399].

Several randomized, double-blind placebo-controlled trials also failed to show the effectiveness of essential fatty acids in the treatment of atopic dermatitis [400,401]. van Gool et al performed a meta-analysis on 22 placebo-controlled studies to examine the potential of oral essential fatty acids to alleviate symptoms of atopic dermatitis [402]. Nineteen studies involved γ-linolenic acid (rich in omega-6 polyunsaturated fatty acids) and five studies involved fish oil supplements (rich in omega-3 polyunsaturated fatty acids) as the intervention (two studies involved both γ-linolenic acid fish oil supplements). The pooled effect size of γ-linolenic acid supplementation on the improvement of the overall severity of atopic dermatitis from 11 trials was 0.15 (95% confidence interval: -0.02 to 0.32). The effect size of fish oil supplementation, calculated from three trials, was even smaller at -0.01 (95% confidence interval: -0.37 to 0.3). For component subscales such as itch, scaling, and lichenification, essential fatty acid supplementation showed no benefit.

Evening primrose oil, derived from the mature seeds of *Oenothera biennis* and contains 10% γ-linolenic acid and 70% linoleic acid may have a beneficial effect in the treatment of atopic dermatitis [133]. A meta-analysis of 26 randomized, double-blind, placebo-controlled clinical trials (n = 1207) showed a statistically significant benefit from evening primrose oil on edema (n = 204; p = 0.0281) and crusting (n = 163; p = 0.0184), and trends in favor of evening primrose oil for most other parameters, particularly itch [403]. The effect usually becomes apparent between 4 and 8 weeks after treatment has been initiated.

Borage oil is an herbal agent with high γ-linolenic acid content. Recently, Foster et al performed a systematic review on 11 clinical trials of oral borage oil (n = 591) and one clinical trial of topical borage oil (n = 100) for the treatment of atopic dermatitis [404]. Additionally, a study on preventive use of borage oil supplementation in neonates at risk of developing atopic dermatitis was included in the analysis. Borage oil contains high levels of omega-6 essential fatty acids and insignificant amounts of omega-3 essential fatty acids [404]. All studies were controlled and most were randomized and double-blind. However, many studies were small and had other methodological limitations. The authors found that the results were highly variable, with the effect reported to be significant in five studies, insignificant in five studies, and mixed in two studies. Borage oil given to at-risk neonates did not prevent development of atopic dermatitis. The authors conclude that nutritional supplementation with borage oil is unlikely to have a major clinical effect but may be useful in some individual patients with less severe atopic dermatitis who are seeking an alternative treatment.

The role of vitamins in the pathogenesis of atopic dermatitis is controversial, suggesting both enhancing and protective mechanisms. An observational study of 138 Norwegian patients (46 males and 92 females) with moderate to severe atopic dermatitis did not find any correlation between low dietary vitamin D intake and clinical disease severity scores [405]. A prospective birth cohort study of 123 6-year-old children showed that atopic dermatitis was more prevalent in the group with higher intake of vitamin D_3[406]. Tsoureli-Nikita et al performed a single-blind clinical trial on 96 subjects (64 males and 32 females; aged 10 to 60 years) with atopic dermatitis [407]. Fifty subjects were given 400 IU of vitamin E of natural origin orally, once a day for 8 months. Forty six subjects took placebo for the same period of time. The authors found that more patients in the placebo group had worse symptoms at the end of the study. The treatment group exhibited a remarkable improvement in facial erythema, lichenification, and the presence of apparently normal skin as well as decreased pruritus. A recent study showed that vitamins E and D supplementation may be beneficial in the treatment of atopic dermatitis [408]. In a double-blind, placebo-controlled study, Javanbakht et al randomized 45 patients aged 13 to 45 years with atopic dermatitis into four groups and treated for 60 days: group P (n = 11), vitamins D and E placebos; group D (n = 12), 1600 IU vitamin D_3 plus vitamin E placebo; group E, 600 IU synthetic all-rac-α-tocopherol plus vitamin D placebo; and group DE (n =11), 1600 IU vitamin D_3plus 600 IU synthetic all-rac-α-tocopherol [408]. The authors found that SCORAD was reduced after 60 days in group D, E, and DE by 34.8%, 35.7%, and 64.3%, respectively (p = 0.004). There was a significant negative association between plasma α-tocopherol and SCORAD, intensity, objective and extent (p = 0.02). More and larger randomized controlled trials are necessary to substantiate these preliminary findings.

A prospective randomized, placebo-controlled trial of 41 adults with atopic dermatitis, Stücker et al showed that topical vitamin B_{12} was superior to placebo with respect to reducing the severity and extent of atopic dermatitis [409]. In this trial, vitamin B_{12}-containing cream was applied to lesions on one side of the body and a placebo preparation on lesions on the contralateral side. Again, more and larger randomized controlled trials are necessary to substantiate this preliminary finding.

In animal studies, flavonoids (vitamin P) have been shown to have a preventative and beneficial effect in mice prone to have atopic dermatitis [410,411]. The preventative effect is dose-dependent and continuous intake of flavonoids significantly decreases the onset and development of atopic dermatitis [410,411]. Data on human studies are scarce. An open trial of 20 adults with atopic dermatitis showed that after a 2- month treatment with a vegetarian diet, the severity of atopic dermatitis was markedly improved as assessed by SCORAD index [412]. Further studies are necessary to substantiate the claim of beneficial effects of flavonoids in the treatment ofatopic dermatitis.

Patient Education

Patient/caregivers education and support are vital in the management of patients with atopic dermatitis. Poor compliance is a major reason for treatment failure [127]. The most important cause is lack of knowledge about the disease and its management [413]. Although there is no cure for atopic dermatitis, control is possible through optimal skin care, avoidance of triggering factors, and pharmacotherapy. Fallacy and misled information may be detrimental to the disease control. Steroid fear or phobia (or its latest variant, tacrolimophobia or pimecrolimophobia) is a significant factor in suboptimal use or non-compliance to treatment [127,132,414,415]. Patients and caregivers should be reassured that topical corticosteroids are safe and effective with their sensible use and they remain the first-line treatment for atopic fares [17]. They need to be taught how to apply topical treatments correctly and in adequate amounts. The International Study of Life with Atopic Dermatitis (ISOLATE) shows that patients with atopic dermatitis are untreated for half the time they are in flare and there is a need for patients to be educated so that they can be confident in using prescribed medication to gain disease control [416]. Studies have shown that age related, structured educational programmes are effective in improving the quality of life of affected children and their caregivers [7,127,417].

Chapter XII

Prognosis

Atopic dermatitis is characterized by exacerbations and remissions. In general, 10-year clearance rates vary from 40 to 80% for those with atopic dermatitis beginning in childhood [263]. Poor prognostic factors include early age at onset, severe disease, family history of atopic dermatitis, and concomitant asthma or allergic rhinitis [102,418]. More than 50% of children with atopic dermatitis subsequently develop of asthma and/or allergic rhinitis in the so-called "atopic march" or "allergic march", particularly in those with early onset, severe and persistent atopic dermatitis [13,19,42,72,75,101].

Chapter XIII

Conclusion

The prevalence of atopic dermatitis is rising dramatically. The disease can adversely influence the quality of care of patients and caregivers and can impose considerable financial impact on the families. Significant advances have been made in our understanding of the pathogenesis. It is hoped that future research will broaden our knowledge in this area so that new treatment strategies can be developed.

References

[1] Leung, AK; Hon, KL; Robson, WL. Atopic dermatitis. *Adv. Pediatr.* 2007;54:241-273.
[2] Leung, AK; Barber, KA. Managing childhood atopic dermatitis. *Adv. Ther.* 2003; 20:129-137.
[3] Leung, AK. Atopic dermatitis. In: Leung, AK. (ed). *Common Problems in Ambulatory Pediatrics.* New York: Nova Science Publishers, Inc., 2011, pp.1325-1336.
[4] Bieber, T. Atopic dermatitis. *Ann. Dermatol.* 2010;22:125-137.
[5] Brenninkmeijer, EE; Legierse, CM; Smitt, JH; et al. The course of life of patients with childhood atopic dermatitis. *Pediatr. Dermatol.* 2009;26:14-22.
[6] Leung, DY; Boguniewicz, M; Howell, MD; et al. New insights into atopic dermatitis. *J. Clin. Invest.* 2004;133:651-657.
[7] Grillo, M; Ng, M; Gassner, L; et al. Pediatric atopic eczema: the impact of an educational intervention. *Pediatr. Dermatol.* 2006;23:428-436.
[8] Cheigh, NH. Managing a common disorder in children: atopic dermatitis. *J. Pediatr. Health Care.* 2003;17:84-88.
[9] Tokura, Y. Extrinsic and intrinsic types of atopic dermatitis. *J. Dermatol. Sci.* 2010;58:1-7.
[10] Bos, JD; Brenninkmeijer, EE; Schram, ME; et al. Atopic eczema or atopiform dermatitis. *Exp. Dermatol.* 2010;19:325-331.
[11] Park, JH; Choi, YL; Namkung, JH; et al. Characteristics of extrinsic vs. intrinsic atopic dermatitis in infancy: correlations with laboratory variables. *Br. J. Dermatol.* 2006;155:778-783.
[12] Boguniewicz, M. Update on atopic dermatitis: insights into pathogenesis and new treatment paradigms. *Allergy Asthma Proc.* 2004;25:279-282.

[13] Dohil, MA; Eichenfield, LF. A treatment approach for atopic dermatitis. *Pediatr. Ann.* 2005; 34:201-210.
[14] Boguniewicz, M; Leung, DYM. Atopic dermatitis. *J. Allergy Clin. Immunol.* 2006;117:S475-480.
[15] Baumer, JH. Atopic eczema in children, NICE. *Arch. Dis. Child. Educ. Pract. Ed.* 2008;93:93-97.
[16] Foroughi, S; Thyagarajan, A; Stone, KD. Advances in pediatric asthma and atopic dermatitis. *Curr. Opin. Pediatr.* 2005;17:658-663.
[17] Krakowski, AC; Eichenfield, L; Dohil, MA. Management of atopic dermatitis in the pediatric population. *Pediatrics.* 2008;122:812-824.
[18] Leung, DY; Nicklas, RA; Li, JT; et al. Disease management of atopic dermatitis: an updated practice parameter. *Ann. Allergy Asthma Immunol.* 2004;93:S1-S21.
[19] Peroni, DG; Piacentini, GL; Bodini, A; et al. Prevalence and risk factors for atopic dermatitis in preschool children. *Br. J. Dermatol.* 2008;158:539-543.
[20] Shaw, TE; Currie, GP; Koudelka, CW; et al. Eczema prevalence in the United States: data from the 2003 National Survey of Children's Health. *J. Invest. Dermatol.* 2011;131:67-73.
[21] Smidesang, I; Saunes, M; Storrø, O; et al. Atopic dermatitis among 2-year olds; high prevalence, but predominately mild disease – the PACT study, Norway. *Pediatr. Dermatol.* 2008;25:13-18.
[22] Asher, MI; Montefort, S; Bjorksten, B; et al. Worldwide time trends in the prevalence of symptoms of asthma, allergic rhinoconjunctivitis, and eczema in childhood: ISAAC phase and three repeat multicountry cross-sectional surveys. *Lancet.* 2006;368:733-743.
[23] Spergel, JM. Epidemiology of atopic dermatitis and atopic march in children. *Immunol. Allergy Clin. North Am.* 2010;30:269-280.
[24] Abramovits, W. Atopic dermatitis. *J. Am. Acad. Dermatol.* 2005; 53:S86-S93.
[25] Simpson, EL; Hanifin, JM. Atopic dermatitis. *J. Am. Acad. Dermatol.* 2005;53:115-128.
[26] Williams, LK; Peterson, EL; Ownby, DR; et al. The relationship between early fever and allergic sensitization at age 6 to 7 years. *J. Allergy Clin. Immunol.* 2004;113:291-296.
[27] Kvenshagen, B; Jacobsen, M; Halvorsen, R. Atopic dermatitis in premature and term children. *Arch. Dis. Child.* 2009;94:202-205.
[28] Leung, TF; Kong, AP; Chan, IH; et al. Association between obesity and atopy in Chinese schoolchildren. *Int. Arch. Allergy Immunol.* 2009;149:133-140.

[29] van Gysel, D; Govaere, E; Verhamme, K; et al. Body mass index in Belgium schoolchildren and its relationship with sensitization and allergic symptoms. *Pediatr. Allergy Immunol.* 2009;20:246-253.
[30] Roos, TC; Geuer, S; Roos, S; et al. Recent advances in treatment strategies for atopic dermatitis. *Drugs.* 2004;64:2639-2666.
[31] Bisgaard, H; Halkjær, LB; Hinge, R; et al. Risk analysis of early childhood eczema. *J. Allergy Clin. Immunol.* 2009;123:1355-1360.
[32] Diepgen, TL; Blettner, M. Analysis of familial aggregation of atopic eczema and other atopic diseases by ODDS RATIO regression models. *J. Invest. Dermatol.* 1996;106:977-981.
[33] Morar, N; Willis-Owen, SAG; Moffatt, MF; et al. The genetics of atopic dermatitis. *J. Allergy Clin. Immunol.* 2006;118:24-34.
[34] Kuster, W; Petersen, M; Christophers, E; et al. A family study of atopic dermatitis. Clinical and genetic characteristics of 188 patients and 2,151 family members. *Arch. Dermatol. Res.* 1990;282:98-102.
[35] Cho, S; Kim, HJ; Oh, SH; et al. The influence of pregnancy and menstruation on the deterioration of atopic dermatitis symptoms. *Ann. Dermatol.* 2010;22:180-185.
[36] Caubet, JC; Eigenmann, PA. Allergic triggers in atopic dermatitis. *Immunol. Allergy Clin. North Am.* 2010;30:289-307.
[37] Epps, RE. Atopic dermatitis and ichthyosis. *Pediatr. Rev.* 2010;31:278-285.
[38] Chien, YH; Hwu, WL; Chiang, BL. The genetics of atopic dermatitis. *Clin. Rev. Allergy Immunol.* 2007;33:178-190.
[39] Schultz Larsen, F. Atopic dermatitis: a genetic-epidemiologic study in a population-based twin sample. *J. Am. Acad. Dermatol.* 1993;28:719-723.
[40] Esparza-Gordillo, J; Weidinger, S; Fölster-Holst, R; et al. A common variant on chromosome 11q13 is associated with atopic dermatitis. *Nat. Genet.* 2009;41:596-601.
[41] Haagerup, A; Bjerke, T; Schiøtz, PO; et al. Atopic dermatitis – a total genome-scan for susceptibility genes. *Acta Derm. Venereol. (Stockh.)* 2004;84:346-352.
[42] Worth, A; Sheikh, A. Food allergy and atopic dermatitis. *Curr. Opin. Allergy Clin. Immunol.* 2010;10:226-230.
[43] Enomoto, H; Hirata, K; Otsuka, K; et al. Filaggrin null mutations are associated with atopic dermatitis and elevated levels of IgE in the Japanese population: a family and case-control study. *J. Hum. Genet.* 2008;53:615-621.

[44] Marenholz, I; Nickel, R; Ruschendorf, F; et al. Filaggrin loss-of-function mutations predispose to phenotypes involved in the atopic march. *J. Allergy Clin. Immunol.* 2006;118:866-871.
[45] Palmer, CN; Irvine, AD; Terron-Kwiatkowski, A; et al. Common loss-of function variants of the epidermal barrier protein filaggrin are a major predisposing factor for atopic dermatitis. *Nat. Genet.* 2006;38:441-446.
[46] van der Oord, RA; Sheikh, A. Filaggrin gene defects and risk of developing allergic sensitisation and allergic disorders: systematic review and meta-analysis. *Br. Med. J.* 2009;339:b2433.
[47] Rodríguez, E; Baurecht, H; Herberich, E; et al. Meta-analysis of filaggrin polymorphisms in eczema and asthma: robust risk factors in atopic disease. *J. Allergy Clin. Immunol.* 2009;123:1361-1370.
[48] Compton, JG; DiGiovanna, JJ; Johnston, KA; et al. Mapping of the associated phenotype of an absent granular in ichthyosis vulgaris to the epidermal differentiation complex on chromosome 1. *Exp. Dermatol.* 2002;11:518-526.
[49] Suh, L. Food allergy and atopic dermatitis: separating fact from friction. *Semin. Cutan. Med. Surg.* 2010;29:72-78.
[50] Ching, GK; Hon, KL; Ng, PC; et al.Filaggrin null mutations in childhood atopic dermatitis among the Chinese.*Int. J. Immunogenet.* 2009 ;36:251-254.
[51] Di Carlo, JB; McCall, CO. Pharmacologic alternatives for severe atopic dermatitis. *Int. J. Dermatol.* 2001;40:82-88.
[52] Leung, DY; Jian, N; Leo, HL. New concepts in the pathogenesis of atopic dermatitis. *Curr. Opin. Immunol.* 2003;15:634-638.
[53] Sugarman, JL; Parish, LC. Efficacy of a lipid-based barrier repair formulation in moderate-to-severe pediatric atopic dermatitis. *J. Drugs. Dermatol.* 2009;8:1106-1111.
[54] de Benedetto, A; Rafaels, NM; McGirt, LY; et al. Tight junction defects in patients with atopic dermatitis. *J. Allergy Clin. Immunol.* 2011;127:773-786.
[55] Ong, PY; Leung, DY. The infectious aspects of atopic dermatitis. *Immunol. Allergy Clin. North Am.* 2010;30:309-321.
[56] Flohr, C; England, K; Radulovic, S; et al. Filaggrin loss-of-function mutations are associated with early-onset eczema, eczema severity and transepidermal water loss at 3 months of age. *Br. J. Dermatol.* 2010;163:1333-1336.
[57] Simpson, E. Are epidermal defects the key initiating factors in the development of atopic dermatitis? *Br. J. Dermatol.* 2010;163:1147-1148.

[58] Leyvraz, C; Charles, RP; Rubera, I; et al. The epidermal barrier function is dependent on the serine protease CAP1/Prss8. *J. Cell. Biol.* 2005;170:487-496.
[59] Nissen, CM. Tight junctions/adherens junctions: basic structure and function. *J. Invest. Dermatol.* 2007;127;2525-2532.
[60] Seidenari, S; Giusti, G. Objective assessmrnt of the skin of children affected by atopic dermatitis: a study of pH, capacitance and TEWL in eczematous and clinically uninvolved skin. *Acta Dermatol. Venereol.* 1995;75:429-433.
[61] Hon, KL; Wong, KY; Leung, TF; et al. Comparison of skin hydration evaluation sites and correlations among skin hydration, transepidermal water loss, SCORAD index, Nottingham Eczema Severity Score, and quality of life in patients with atopic dermatitis. *Am. J. Clin. Dermatol.* 2008;9:45-50.
[62] Nemoto-Hasebe, I; Akiyama, M; Nomura, T; et al. Clinical severity correlates with impaired barrier in filaggrin-related eczema. *J. Invest. Dermatol.* 2009;129:682-689.
[63] Candi, E; Schmidt, R; Melino, G. The cornified envelope: a model of cell death in the skin. *Nat. Rev. Mol. Cell Biol.* 2005;6:328-340.
[64] Wollenberg, A; Schnopp, C. Evolution of conventional therapy in atopic dermatitis. *Immunol. Allergy Clin. North Am.* 2010;30:351-368.
[65] Hara, J; Higuchi, K; Okamoto, R; et al. High-expression of sphingomyelin deacylase is an important determinant of ceramide deficiency leading to barrier disruption in atopic dermatitis. *J. Invest. Dermatol.* 2000;115:406-413.
[66] Imokawa, G. Lipid abnormalities in atopic dermatitis. *J. Am. Acad. Dermatol.* 2001;45(suppl):S29-S32.
[67] Beltrani, VS; Boguneiwicz, M. Atopic dermatitis. *Dermatol. Online J.* 2003; 9(2): 1.
[68] Sator, PG; Schmidt, JB; Hönigsmann, H. Comparison of epidermal hydration and skin surface lipids in healthy individuals and in patients with atopic dermatitis. *J. Am. Acad. Dermatol.* 2003;48:352-358.
[69] Ong, PY; Ohtake, T; Brandt, C; et al. Endogenous antimicrobial peptides and skin infections in atopic dermatitis. *N. Engl. J. Med.* 2002;347:1151-1160.
[70] Schluter, H; Moll, I; Wolburg,H; et al. The different structures containing tight junction proteins in epidermal and other stratified epithelial cells, including squamous cell metaplasia. *Eur. J. Cell Biol.* 2007;86:645-655.
[71] van Itallie, CM; Anderson, JM. Claudins and epithelial paracellular transport. *Ann. Rev. Physiol.* 2006;68:403-429.

[72] Boguniewicz, M; Eichenfield, LF; Hultsch, T. Current management of atopic dermatitis and interruption of the atopic march. *J. Allergy Clin. Immunol.* 2003;112:S140-S149.
[73] Huang, JT; Abrams, M; Tlougan, B; et al. Treatment of *Staphylococcus aureus* colonization in atopic dermatitis decreases disease severity. *Pediatrics*. 2009;123:e808-e814.
[74] Cho, SH; Strickland, I; Boguniewicz, M; et al. Fibronectin and fibrinogen contribute to the enhanced binding of *Staphylococcus aureus* to atopic skin. *J. Allergy Clin. Immunol.* 2001;108:269-274.
[75] Traidl-Hoffman, C; Mempel, M; Belloni, B; et al. Therapeutic management of atopic dermatitis. *Curr. Drug Metab.* 2010;11:234-241.
[76] Suh, L; Coffin, S; Leckerman, KH; et al. Methicillin-resistant *Staphylococcus aureus* colonization in children with atopic dermatitis. *Pediatr. Dermatol.* 2008;25:528-534.
[77] Chiu, LS; Chow, VC; Ling, JM; et al. *Staphylococcus aureus* carriage in the anterior nares of close contacts of patients with atopic dermatitis. *Arch. Dermatol.* 2010;146:748-752.
[78] Bonness, S; Szekat, C; Novak, N; et al. Pulsed-field gel electrophoresis of *Staphylococcus aureus* isolates from atopic patients revealing presence of similar strains in isolates from children and their parents. *J. Clin. Microbiol.* 2008;46:456-461.
[79] Chiu, LS; Ho, MS; Hsu, LY; et al. Prevalence and molecular characteristics of *Staphylococcus aureus* isolates colonizing patients with atopic dermatitis and their close contacts in Singapore. *Br. J. Dermatol.* 2009;160:965-971.
[80] Leung, DY. Infection in atopic dermatitis. *Curr. Opin. Pediatr.* 2003;15:399-404.
[81] Krakowski, AC; Dohil, MA. Topical therapy in pediatric atopic dermatitis. *Semin. Cutan. Med. Surg.* 2008;27:161-167.
[82] Breuer, K; Haussler, S; Kapp, A; et al. *Staphylococcus aureus*: colonizing features and influence of an antibacterial treatment in adults with atopic dermatitis. *Br. J. Dermatol.* 2002;147:55-61.
[83] Baker, BS. The role of microorganisms in atopic dermatitis. *Clin. Exp. Immunol.* 2006; 114:1-9.
[84] Ong, PY; Patel, M; Ferdman, RM; et al. Association of staphylococcal superantigen-specific immunoglobulin E with mild and moderate atopic dermatitis. *J. Pediatr.* 2008;153:803-806.
[85] Tomi, NS; Kranke, B; Aberer, E. Staphylococcal toxins in patients with psoriasis, atopic dermatitis, and erythroderma, and healthy control subjects. *J. Am. Acad. Dermatol.* 2005;53:67-72.

[86] Leung, DY; Hanifin, JM; Pariser, DM; et al. Effects of pimecrolimus cream 1% in the treatment of patients with atopic dermatitis who demonstrate a clinical insensitivity to topical corticosteroids: a randomized, multicentre vehicle-controlled trial. *Br. J. Dermatol.* 2009;161:435-443.

[87] Wedi, B; Wieczorek, D; Stünkel, T; et al. Staphylococcal exotoxins exert proinflammatory effects through inhibition of eosinophil apoptosis, increased surface antigen expression (CD11b, CD45, CD54, and CD69), and enhanced cytokine-activated oxidative burst, thereby triggering allergic inflammatory reactions. *J. Allergy Clin. Immunol.* 2002;109:477-484.

[88] Bunikowski, R; Mielke, M; Skarabis, H; et al. Prevalence and role of serum IgE antibodies to the *Staphylococcus aureus*-derived superantigens SEA and SEB in children with atopic dermatitis. *J. Allergy Clin. Immunol.* 1999;103:119-124.

[89] Hofer, MF; Harbeck, RJ; Schlievert, PM; et al. Staphylococcal toxins augment specific IgE responses by atopic patients exposed to allergen. *J. Invest. Dermatol.* 1999;112:171-176.

[90] Hauk, PJ; Hamid, QA; Chrousos, GP; et al. Induction of corticosteroid insensitivity in human PBMCs by microbial superantigens. *J. Allergy Clin. Immunol.* 2000;105:782-787.

[91] Li, LB; Goleva, E; Hall, CF; et al. Superantigen-induced corticosteroid resistance of human T cells occurs through activation of the mitogen-activated protein kinase/extracellular signal-regulated kinase (MEK-ERK) pathway. *J. Allergy Clin. Immunol.* 2004;114:1059-1069.

[92] Karasuyama, H; Mukai, K; Tsujimura, Y; et al. Newly discovered roles for basophils: a neglected minority gains new respect. *Nat. Rev. Immunol.* 2009;9:9-13.

[93] Gong, JQ; Lin, L; Lin, T; et al. Skin colonization by *Staphylococcus aureus* in patients with eczema and atopic dermatitis and relevant combined topical therapy: a double-blind multicentre randomized controlled trial. *Br. J. Dermatol.* 2006;155:680-687.

[94] Gilani, SJ; Gonzalez, M; Hussain, I; et al. *Staphylococcus aureus* re-colonization in atopic eczema: beyond the skin. *Clin. Exp. Dermatol.* 2005;30:10-13.

[95] Travers, JB; Kozman, A; Mousdicas, N; et al. Infected atopic dermatitis lesions contain pharmacologic amounts of lipoteichoic acid. *J. Allergy Clin. Immunol.* 2010;125:146-152.

[96] Sugita, T; Suto, H; Unno, T; et al. Molecular analysis of *Malassezia* microflora on the skin of atopic dermatitis patients and healthy subjects. *J. Clin. Microbiol.* 2001;39:3486-3490.

[97] Sugita, T; Tajima, M; Tsubuku, H; et al. Quantitative analysis of cutaneous *Malassezia* in atopic dermatitis patients using real-time PCR. *Microbiol. Immunol.* 2006;50:549-552.
[98] Wessels, MW; Doeks, G; van Ieperen-van Dijk, AG; et al. IgE antibodies to *Pityrosporonovale* in atopic dermatitis. *Br. J. Dermatol.* 1991;125:227-232.
[99] Buentke, E; Scheynius, A. Dendritic cells and fungi. *APMIS.* 2003;111:789-796.
[100] Wong, AW; Hon, EK; Zee, B. Is topical antimycotic treatment useful as adjuvant therapy for flexural atopic dermatitis: randomized, double-blind, controlled trial using one side of the elbow or knee as a control?*Int. J. Dermatol.*2008;47:187-191.
[101] Plötz, SG; Ring, J. What's new in atopic eczema? *Expert Opin. Emerg. Drugs.* 2010;15:249-267.
[102] Levy, RM; Gelfand, JM; Yan, AC. The epidemiology of atopic dermatitis. *Clin. Dermatol.* 2003;21:109-115.
[103] Kalliomäki, M; Salminen, S; Poussa, T; et al. Probiotics and prevention of atopic disease: 4-year follow-up of a randomised placebo-controlled trial. *Lancet.* 2003;361:1869-1871.
[104] Watanabe, S; Narisawa, Y; Arase, S; et al. Differences in fecal microflora between patients with atopic dermatitis and healthy control subjects. *J. Allergy Clin. Immunol.* 2003;111:587-591.
[105] Schmitt, J; Schmitt, NM; Kirch, W; et al. Early exposure to antibiotics and infections and the incidence of atopic eczema: a population-based cohort study. *Pediatr. Allergy Immunol.* 2010;21:292-300.
[106] Munoz-Hoyos, A; Espin-Quirantes, C; Molina-Carballo, A; et al. Neuroendocrine and circadian aspects (melatonin and β-endorphin) of atopic dermatitis in the child. *Pediatr. Allergy Immunol.* 2007;18:679-686.
[107] Hon, KL; Lam, MC; Wong, KY; et al. Pathophysiology of nocturnal scratching in childhood atopic dermatitis: the role of brain-derived neurotrophic factor and substance P. *Br. J. Dermatol.* 2007;157:922-925.
[108] Raap, U; Goltz, C; Deneka, N; et al. Brain-derived neurotrophic factor is increased in atopic dermatitis and modulates eosinophil functions compared with that seen in nonatopic subjects. *J. Allergy Clin. Immunol.* 2005;115:1268-1275.
[109] Kim, JS. Pediatric atopic dermatitis: the importance of food allergens. *Semin. Cutan. Med. Surg.* 2008;27:156-160.
[110] Leung, AK. Food allergy: a clinical approach. *Adv. Pediatr.* 1998;45:145-177.

[111] Werfel, T; Breuer, K. Role of food allergy in atopic dermatitis. *Curr. Opin. Allergy Clin. Immunol.* 2004;4:379-385.
[112] Greenhawt, M. The role of food allergy in atopic dermatitis. *Allergy Asthma Proc.* 2010;31:392-397.
[113] Sampson, HA. The immunopathogenic role of food hypersensitivity in atopic dermatitis. *Acta Derm. Venereol.* 1992;176(Suppl):534-557.
[114] Burks, AW; Mallroy, SB; Williams, LW; et al. Atopic dermatitis: clinical relevance of food hypersensitivity reactions. *J. Pediatr.* 1988;113:447-451.
[115] Hoffman, KM; Sampson, HA. Evaluation and management of patients with adverse food reactions. In: Bierman, CW; Pearlman, DS; Shapiro, GG; et al. (eds). *Allergy, asthma, and immunology from infancy to adulthood.* Philadelphia: W.B. Saunders, 1999, pp.665-686.
[116] Sampson, HA. Food sensitivity and the pathogenesis of atopic dermatitis. *J. R. Soc. Med.* 1997;90:2-8.
[117] Breuer, K; Heratizadeh, A; Wulf, A; et al. Late eczematous reactions to food in children with atopic dermatitis. *Clin. Exp. Allergy.* 2004;34:817-824.
[118] Hill, DJ; Hosking, CS. Food allergy and atopic dermatitis in infancy: an epidemiologic study. *Pediatr. Allergy Immunol.* 2004;15:421-427.
[119] Leung, AK; Bowen, TJ. Seasonal allergic rhinitis and food allergy. In: Bergman, AB. (ed). *Twenty Common Problems in Pediatrics.* New York: McGraw-Hill, 2001, pp.219-233.
[120] Hon, KL; Chan, IH; Chow, CM; et al. Specific IgE of common foods in Chinese children with eczema.*Pediatr. Allergy Immunol.* 2011;22:50-53.
[121] Langan, SM; Silcocks, P; Williams, HC. What causes flares of eczema in children? *Br. J. Dermatol.* 2009;161:640-646.
[122] Sicherer, SH; Leung, DY. Advances in allergic skin disease, anaphylaxis, and hypersensitivity reactions to foods, drugs, and insects. *J. Allergy Clin. Immunol.* 2007;119:1462-1469.
[123] Shek, LP; Chong, AR; Soh, SE; et al. Specific profiles of house dust mite sensitization in children with asthma and in children with eczema. *Pediatr. Allergy Immunol.* 2010;21:e718-e722.
[124] Novak, N; Allam, JP; Bieber, T. Allergic hyperreactivity to microbial components: a trigger factor of "intrinsic" atopic dermatitis? *J. Allergy Clin. Immunol.* 2003;112:215-216.
[125] Tupker, RA; De Monchy, JGR; Coenraads, PJ; et al. Induction of atopic dermatitis by inhalation of house dust mite. *J. Allergy Clin. Immunol.* 1996;97:1064-1070.

[126] Böhme, M; Kull, I; Bergström, A; et al. Parental smoking increases the risk for eczema with sensitization in 4-year-old children. *J. Allergy Clin. Immunol.* 2010;125:941-943.
[127] Kienast, AK; Hoeger, PH. Atopic dermatitis in children: what to do when nothing works. *G. Ital. Dermatol. Venereol.* 2010;145:303-308.
[128] Krämer, U; Lemmen, CH; Behrendt, H; et al. The effect of environmental tobacco smoke on eczema and allergic sensitization in children. *Br. J. Dermatol.* 2004;150:111-118.
[129] Sturgill, S; Bernard, LA. Atopic dermatitis update. *Curr. Opin. Pediatr.* 2004;16:396-401.
[130] Hon, KL; Ching, GK; Hung, EC; et al. Serum lead levels in childhood eczema.*Clin. Exp. Dermatol.* 2009;34:e508-e509.
[131] Hon, KL; Wang, SS; Hung, EC; et al. Serum levels of heavy metals in childhood eczema and skin diseases: friends or foes. *Pediatr. Allergy Immunol.* 2010;21:831-836.
[132] Anderson, PC; Dinulos, JG. Atopic dermatitis and alternative management strategies. *Curr. Opin. Pediatr.* 2009;21:131-138.
[133] Finch, J; Munhutu, MN; Whitaker-Worth, DL. Atopic dermatitis and nutrition. *Clin. Dermatol.* 2010;28:605-614.
[134] Darsow, U; Lübbe, J; Taïab, A; et al. Position paper on diagnosis and treatment of atopic dermatitis. *J. Eur. Acad. Dermatol. Venereol.* 2005;19:286-295.
[135] Manzini, BM; Ferdani, G; Simonetti, V; et al. Contact sensitization in children. *Contact Dermatitis.* 1998;15:12-17.
[136] Mortz, CG; Andersen, KE. Allergic contact dermatitis in children and adolescents. *Contact Dermatitis.* 1999;41:121-130.
[137] Schmid-Ott, G; Jaeger, B; Meyer, S; et al. Different expression of cytokine and membrane molecules by circulating lymphocytes on acute mental stress in patients with atopic dermatitis in comparison with healthy controls. *J. Allergy Clin. Immunol.* 2001;108:455-462.
[138] Akdis, CA; Akdi, M; Bieber, T; et al. Diagnosis and treatment of atopic dermatitis in children and adults: European Academy of Allergology and Clinical Immunology/American Academy of Allergy, Asthma and Immunology/PRACTALL Consensus Report. *J. Allergy Clin. Immunol.* 2006;118:152-169.
[139] Salomon, J; Baran, E. The role of selected neuropeptides in pathogenesis of atopic dermatitis. *J. Eur. Acad. Dermatol. Venereol.* 2008;22:223-228.
[140] Kobaly, K; Somani, AK; McCormick, T; et al. Effects of occlusion on the skin of atopic dermatitis patients. *Dermatitis.* 2010;21:255-261.

[141] Beltrani, VS. Suggestions regarding a more appropriate understanding of atopic dermatitis. *Curr. Opin. Allergy Clin. Immunol.* 2005;5:413-418.
[142] Potapova, OV; Luzgina, NG; Shkurupiy, VA. Immunomorphological study of Langerhans cells in the skin of patients with atopic dermatitis. *Bull. Exp. Biol. Med.* 2008;146:809-811.
[143] Rudikoff, D; Lebwohl, M. Atopic dermatitis. *Lancet.* 1998;351:1715-1721.
[144] Darsow, U; Pfab, F; Valet, M; et al. Pruritus and atopic dermatitis. *Clin. Rev. Allergy Immunol.* (in press).
[145] Gutzmer, R; Mommert, S; Gschwandtner, M; et al. The histamine H4 receptor is functionally expressed on Th2 cells. *J. Allergy Clin. Immunol.* 2009;123:619-625.
[146] Kristal, L; Klein, PA. Atopic dermatitis in infants and children. *Pediatr. Clin. North Am.* 2000;47:877-895.
[147] Halkjær, LB; Loland, L; Buchvald, FF; et al. Development of atopic dermatitis during the first 3 years of life: the Copenhagen Prospective Study on Asthma in Childhood cohort study in high-risk children. *Arch. Dermatol.* 2006;142:561-566.
[148] Eigenmann, PA. Clinical features and diagnostic criteria of atopic dermatitis in relation to age. *Pediatr. Allergy Immunol.* 2001;12(Suppl 14):69-74.
[149] Hanifin, JM. Atopic dermatitis. *J. Am. Acad. Dermatol.* 1982;6:1-13.
[150] Leung, AK; Feingold, M. Pityriasis alba. *AJDC.* 1986;140:379-380.
[151] Leung, AK; Kao, CP. Keratosis pilaris. *Consultant Pediatrician.* 2004;3:188-191.
[152] Leung, AK; Robson, WL. Ichthyosis vulgaris. *Consultant Pediatrician.* 2006;5:573-575.
[153] Kang, K; Polster, AM; Nedorost, S; et al. Atopic dermatitis. In: Bolognia, JL; Jorizzo, JL; Rapini, RP. (eds). *Dermatology.* Philadelphia: Mosby, 2003, pp.199-214.
[154] Krafchik, BR; Halbert, A; Yamamoto, K; et al. Atopic dermatitis. In: Schachner, LA; Hansen, RC; Happle, R; et al. (eds). *Pediatric Dermatology.* 3rd edition. Philadelphia: Mosby, 2003, pp.599-630.
[155] Hanifin, JM; Rajka, G. Diagnostic features of atopic dermatitis. *Acta Derm. Venereol. (Stockh.)* 1980;92(Suppl):44-47.
[156] Böhme, M; Svensson, A; Kull, I; et al. Hanifin's and Rajka's minor criteria for atopic dermatitis. Which do 2-year-olds exhibit? *J. Am. Acad. Dermatol.* 2000;43:285-292.
[157] Nagaraja, Kanwar, AJ; Dhar, S; Singh, S; et al. Frequency and significance of minor clinical features in various age-related subgroups of atopic dermatitis in children. *Pediatr. Dermatol.* 1996;13:10-13.

[158] Williams, HC; Burney, PG; Pembroke, AC; et al. The U.K. Working Party's diagnostic criteria for atopic dermatitis, III: independent hospital validation. *Br. J. Dermatol.* 1994;131:406-416.
[159] Eichenfield, LF; Hanifin, JM; Luger, TA; et al. Consensus conference on pediatric AD. *J. Am. Acad. Dermatol.* 2003;49:1088-1095.
[160] Eichenfield, LF. Consensus guidelines in diagnosis and treatment of atopic dermatitis. *Allergy.* 2004;59(Suppl 78):86-92.
[161] European Task Force on Atopic dermatitis. Severity scoring of atopic dermatitis: the SCORAD index. Consensus Report of the European Task Force on atopic dermatitis. *Dermatology.* 1993;186-23-31.
[162] Hon, KLE; Leung, TF; Wong, Y; et al. Lesson from performing SCORADs in children with atopic dermatitis: subjective symptoms do not correlate well with disease extent or intensity. *Int. J. Dermatol.* 2006;45:728-730.
[163] Kunz, B; Oranje, AP; Labrèze, L; et al. Clinical validation and guidelines for the SCORAD Index: consensus report of the European Task Force on Atopic dermatitis. *Dermatology.* 1997;195:10-19.
[164] Benjamin, K; Waterston, K; Russell, M; et al. The development of an objective method for measuring scratch in children with atopic dermatitis suitable for clinical use. *J. Am. Acad. Dermatol.* 2004;50:33-40.
[165] Hon, KLE; Lam, MCA; Leung, TF; et al. Nocturnal wrist movements are correlated with objective clinical scores and plasma chemokine levels in children with atopic dermatitis. *Br. J. Dermatol.* 2006;154:629-635.
[166] Hon, KLE; Lam, MCA; Leung, TF; et al. Nocturnal wrist movements are correlated with objective clinical scores and plasma chemokine levels in children with atopic dermatitis. *Br. J. Dermatol.* 2006b;154:629-635.
[167] Kawada, T. Monitoring of activity by wrist accelerometer in patients with atopic dermatitis. *Clin. Exp. Dermatol.* 2009;35:193-208.
[168] Hon, KLE; Leung, TF; Ma, KC; et al. Resting energy expenditure, oxygen consumption and carbon dioxide production during sleep in children with atopic dermatitis. *J. Dermatol. Treat.* 2005;16:22-25.
[169] Hanifin, JM; Thurston, M; Omoto, M; et al. The eczema area and severity index (EASI): assessment of reliability in atopic dermatitis. EASI Evaluator Group. *Exp. Dermatol.* 2001;10:11-18.
[170] Emerson, RM; Charman, CR; Williams, HC. The Nottingham Eczema Severity Score: preliminary refinement of the Rajka and Langeland grading. *Br. J. Dermatol.* 2000;142:288-297.
[171] Hon, KLE; Ma, KC; Wong, E; et al. Validation of a self-administered questionnaire in Chinese in the assessment of eczema severity. *Pediatr. Dermatol.* 2003;20:465-469.

[172] Leung, TF; Ma, KC; Hon, KL; et al. Serum concentration of macrophage-derived chemokine may be a useful inflammatory marker for assessing severity of atopic dermatitis in infants and young children. *Pediatr. Allergy Immunol.* 2003;14:296-301.

[173] Hon, KLE; Leung, TF; Ma, KC; et al. Serum levels of cutaneous T-cell attracting chemokine (CTACK) as a laboratory marker of the severity of atopic dermatitis in children. *Clin. Exp. Dermatol.* 2004;29:293-296.

[174] Hon, KLE; Leung, TF; Ma, KC; et al. Urinary leukotriene E4 correlates with severity of atopic dermatitis in children. *Clin. Exp. Dermatol.* 2004;29:277-281.

[175] Hon, KLE; Leung, TF; Ma, KC; et al. Serum concentration of IL-18 correlates with disease extent in young children with atopic dermatitis. *Pediatr. Dermatol.* 2004;21:619-622.

[176] Leung, TF; Wong, CK; Chan, IH; et al. Plasma concentration of thymus and activation-regulated chemokine is elevated in childhood asthma. *J. Allergy Clin. Immunol.* 2002;110:404-409.

[177] Leung, TF; Wong, CK; Lam, CWK; et al. Plasma TARC concentration may be a useful marker for asthmatic exacerbation in children. *Eur. Respir. J.* 2003;21:616-620.

[178] Morales, J; Homey, B; Vicari, AP; et al. CTACK, a skin-associated chemokine that preferentially attracts skin-homing memory T cells. *Proc. Natl. Acad. Sci. USA*. 1999;96:14470-14475.

[179] Hon, KL; Leung, TF; Wong, KY; et al. Does age or gender influence quality of life in children with atopic dermatitis? *Clin. Exp. Dermatol.* 2008;33:705-709.

[180] Hon, KL; Leung, TF. Seromarkers in childhood atopic dermatitis. *Expert Rev. Dermatol.* 2010;5:299-314.

[181] Hon, KL; Chan, HI; Chow, CM; et al. Exploring CCL18, eczema severity and atopy. *Pediatr. Allergy Immunol.* (in press).

[182] Ben-Gashir, MA; Seed, PT; Hay, RJ. Quality of life and disease severity are correlated in children with atopic dermatitis. *Br. J. Dermatol.* 2004;150:284-290.

[183] Holm, EA; Wulf, HC; Stegmann, H; et al. Life quality assessment among patients with atopic eczema. *Br. J. Dermatol.* 2006;154:719-725.

[184] Lewis-Jones, MS; Finlay, AY. The Children's Dermatology Life Quality Index (CDLQI): initial validation and practical use. *Br. J. Dermatol.* 1995;132:942-949.

[185] Chamlin, SL; Cella, D; Frieden, IJ; et al. Development of the childhood atopic dermatitis impact scale: initial validation of a quality-of-life measure

for young children with atopic dermatitis and their families. *J. Invest. Dermatol.* 2005;125:1106-1111.
[186] McKenna, SP; Doward, LC. Quality of life of children with atopic dermatitis and their families. *Curr. Opin. Allergy Clin. Immunol.* 2008;8:228-231.
[187] McKenna, SP; Whalley, D; Dewar, AL; et al. International development of the Parents' Index of Quality of Life in Atopic Dermatitis (PIQoL-AD). *Qual. Life Res.* 2005;14:231-241.
[188] Meads, DM; McKenna, SP; Kahler, K. The quality of life of parents of children with atopic dermatitis: interpretation of PIQoL-AD scores. *Qual. Life Res.* 2005;14:2235-2245.
[189] Drake, L; Prendergast, M; Maher, R; et al. The impact of tacrolimus ointment on health-related quality of life of adult and pediatric patients with atopic dermatitis. *J. Am. Acad. Dermatol.* 2001;44:S65-S72.
[190] Whalley, D; Huels, J; McKenna, SP; et al. The benefit of pimecrolimus (Elidel, SDZ ASM 981) on parents' quality of life in the treatment of pediatric atopic dermatitis. *Pediatrics.* 2002;110:1133113-6.
[191] Krol, A; Krafchik, B. The differential diagnosis of atopic dermatitis in childhood. *Dermatol. Ther.* 2006;19:73-82.
[192] Leung, AK; Robson, WL. Psoriasis. *Consultant.* 2005;45:578-579.
[193] Leung, AKC; Robson, WL. Nummular eczema (discoid eczema). *Consultant Pediatrician.* 2006;5:790-793.
[194] Leung, AK; Martin, S. Drug therapy for some common pediatric skin eruptions. *Drug Protocol.* 1987;2:9-20.
[195] Hon, KLE; Lam, MCA; Leung, TF; et al. Clinical features associated with nasal *Staphylococcus aureus* colonization in Chinese children with moderate-to-severe atopic dermatitis. *Ann. Acad. Med. Singapore.* 2005;34:602-605.
[196] Farajzadeh, S; Rahnama, Z; Kamyabi, Z; et al. Bacterial colonization and antibiotic resistance in children with atopic dermatitis. *Dermatol. Online J.* 2008;14(7):21.
[197] Hon, KL; Leung, AK; Kong, AY; et al. Atopic dermatitis complicated with methicillin-resistant *Staphylococcus aureus* infection. *J. Natl. Med. Assoc.* 2008;100:797-800.
[198] Hayakawa, K; Hirahara, K; Fukuda, T; et al. Risk factors for severe impetiginized atopic dermatitis in Japan and assessment of its microbiological features. *Clin. Exp. Dermatol.* 2009;34:e63-e65.

[199] Park, JM; Oh, SH; Kim, J; et al. Atopic dermatitis with group A beta-hemolytic Streptococcus skin infection complicated by posterior reversible encephalopathy syndrome. *Arch. Dermatol.* 2009;145:846-847.
[200] Babic, MJ. Eczema vaccinatum: a reaction to the smallpox vaccine. *Am. J. Nurs.* 2007;107:30-31.
[201] Bair, B; Dodd, J; Heidelberg, K; et al. Cataracts in atopic dermatitis. A case presentation and review of the literature. *Arch. Dermatol.* (in press).
[202] Bielory, B; Bielory, L. Atopic dermatitis and keratoconjunctivitis. *Immunol. Allergy Clin. North Am.* 2010;30:323-336.
[203] Sidbury, R; Poorsattar, S. Pediatric atopic dermatitis: should we treat it differently? *Dermatol. Ther.* 2006;19:83-90.
[204] Chamlin, SL; Frieden, IJ; Williams, ML; et al. Effects of atopic dermatitis on young American children and their families. *Pediatrics.* 2004;114:607-611.
[205] Chamlin, SL; Chren, MM. Quality-of-life outcomes and measurement in childhood atopic dermatitis. *Immunol. Allergy Clin. North Am.* 2010;30:281-288.
[206] Dennis, H; Rostill, H; Reed, J; et al. Factors promoting psychological adjustment to childhood atopic eczema. *J. Child Health Care.* 2006;10:126-139.
[207] Kelsay, K. Addressing psychological aspects of atopic dermatitis. *Immunol. Allergy Clin. North Am.* 2010;30:385-396.
[208] Kelsay, K. Management of sleep disturbance associated with atopic dermatitis. *J. Allergy Clin. Immunol.* 2006;118:198-201.
[209] Ricci, G; Dondi, A; Patrizi, A; et al. Systemic therapy of atopic dermatitis in children. *Drugs.* 2009;69:297-306.
[210] Shani-Adir, A; Rozenman, D; Kessel, A; et al. The relationship between sensory hypersensitivity and sleep quality of children with atopic dermatitis. *Pediatr. Dermatol.* 2009;26:143-149.
[211] Hon, KL; Kam, WY; Lam, MC; et al. CDLQI, SCORAD and NESS: are they correlated? *Qual. Life Res.* 2006;15:1551-1558.
[212] Weisshaar, E; Diepgen, TL; Bruckner, T; et al. Itch intensity evaluated in the German Atopic Dermatitis Intervention Study (GADIS): correlations with quality of life, coping behavior and SCORAD severity in 823 children. *Acta Derm. Venereol.* 2008;88:234-230.
[213] Carroll, CL; Balkrishnan, R; Feldman, SR; et al. The burden of atopic dermatitis: impact on the patient, family, and society. *Pediatr. Dermatol.* 2005;22:192-199.

[214] Chamlin, SL. The psychosocial burden of childhood atopic dermatitis. *Dermatol. Ther.* 2006;19:104-107.
[215] Kiebert, G; Sorensen, SV; Revicki, D; et al. Atopic dermatitis is associated with a decrement in health-related quality of life. *Int. J. Dermatol.* 2002;41:151-158.
[216] Faught, J; Bierl, C; Barton, B; et al. Stress in mothers of young children with eczema. *Arch. Dis. Child.* 2007;92:683-686.
[217] Al Shobaili, HA. The impact of childhood atopic dermatitis on the patients' family. *Pediatr. Dermatol.* 2010;27:618-623.
[218] Moore, K; David, T; Murray, C; et al. Effect of childhood eczema and asthma on parental sleep and well-being: a prospective comparative study. *Br. J. Dermatol.* 2006;154:514-518.
[219] Warschburger, P; Buchholz, HT; Petermann, F. Psychological adjustment in parents of young children with atopic dermatitis: which factors predict parental quality of life.*Br. J. Dermatol.* 2004;150:304-311.
[220] Alvarenga, T; Calddeira, A. Quality of life in pediatric patients with atopic dermatitis. *J. Pediatr. (Rio J.)* 2009;85:415-420.
[221] Chamlin, SL; Mattson, CL; Frieden, IJ; et al. The price of pruritus: sleep disturbance and cosleeping in atopic dermatitis. *Arch. Pediatr. Adolesc. Med.* 2005;159:745-750.
[222] Mancini, A; Kaulback, K; Chamlin, SL; et al. The socioeconomic impact of atopic dermatitis in the United States: a systematic review. *Pediatr. Dermatol.* 2008;25:1-6.
[223] Taïeb, A. Allergy workup: when and how for the child with atopic dermatitis? *Acta Derm. Venereol.* 2005; 215(Suppl):16-20.
[224] Hon, KL; Ching, GK; Wong, KY; et al. A pilot study to explore the usefulness of antibody array in childhood atopic dermatitis. *J. Natl. Med. Assoc.* 2008;100:500-504.
[225] Bingham, EA. Guidelines to management of atopic dermatitis. In: Harper, J; Oranje, A; Prose N. (eds). *Textbook of Pediatric Dermatology.* 2nd edition. Oxford: Blackwell Publishing, 2006, pp.259-275.
[226] Wahn, U; Warner, J; Simons, FE; et al. IgE antibody responses in young children with atopic dermatitis. *Pediatr. Allergy Immunol.* 2008;19:332-336.
[227] Breneman, D; Fleischer, A, Jr.; Abramovits, W; et al. Intermittent therapy for flare prevention and long-term disease control in stabilized atopic dermatitis: a randomized comparison of 3-times-weekly applications of tacrolimus ointment versus vehicle. *J. Am. Acad. Dermatol.* 2008;58:990-999.

[228] Brenninkmeijer, EE; Spuls, PI; Legierse, CM; et al. Clinical differences between atopic and atopiform dermatitis. *J. Am. Acad. Dermatol.* 2008;58:407-414.

[229] Opper, FH; Burakoff, R. Food allergy and intolerance. *Gastroenterologist.* 1993;1:211-220.

[230] Boguniewicz, M; Schmid-Grendelmeier, P; Leung, DYM. Atopic dermatitis. *J. Allergy Clin. Immunol.* 2006;118:40-43.

[231] Boguniewicz, M; Zeichner,JA; Eichenfield, LF; et al. MAS063DP is effective monotherapy for mild to moderate atopic dermatitis in infants and children: a multicenter, randomized, vehicle-controlled study. *J. Pediatr.* 2008;152:854-859.

[232] Bock, SA; Atkins, FM. Patterns of food hypersensitivity during sixteen years of double-blind, placebo-controlled food challenges. *J. Pediatr.* 1990;117:561-567.

[233] Nosbaum, A; Hennino, A; Berard, F; et al. Patch testing in atopic dermatitis patients. *Eur. J. Dermatol.* 2010;20:563-566.

[234] Kerschenlohr, K; Darsow, U; Burgdorf, WHC; et al. Lessons from atopy patch testing in atopic dermatitis. *Curr. Allergy Asthma Rep.* 2004;4:285-289.

[235] Lipozenčić, J; Wolf, R. The diagnostic value of atopy patch testing and prick testing in atopic dermatitis: facts and controversies. *Clin. Dermatol.* 2010;28:38-44.

[236] Turjanmaa, K; Darsow, U; Niggemann, B; et al. EAACI/GA2LEN position paper: present status of the atopy patch test. *Allergy.* 2006;61:1377-1384.

[237] Shaw, JC. Atopic dermatitis (eczema). In: Rose, RD. (ed). *UpToDate.* Waltham, MA, 2006.

[238] Shaw, MG; Burkhart, CN; Morrell, DS. Systemic therapies for pediatric atopic dermatitis: a review for the primary care physician. *Pediatr. Ann.* 2009;38:380-387.

[239] Schäfer, T; Borowski, C; Reese, I; et al. Systematic review and evidence-based consensus guideline on prevention of allergy and atopic eczema of the German Network on Allergy Prevention (ABAP). *Minerva Pediatr.* 2008;60:313-325.

[240] Schäfer, T; Stieger, B; Polzius, R. Atopic eczema and indoor climate: results from the children from Lübeck allergy and environment study (KLAUS). *Allergy.* 2008;63:244-246.

[241] Sampson, HA; McCaskill, CC. Food hypersensitivity and atopic dermatitis: evaluation of 113 patients. *J. Pediatr.* 1985;107:669-675.

[242] Bath-Hextall, FJ; Delamere, FM; Williams, HC.Dietary exclusions for established atopic eczema.*Cochrane Database Syst. Rev.*2008;(1):CD005203.
[243] Bath-Hextall, FJ; Delamere, FM; Williams, HC.Dietary exclusions for improving established atopic eczema in adults and children: systematic review.*Allergy*.2009;64:258-264.
[244] Batchelor, JM; Grindlay, DJ; Williams, HC.What's new in atopic eczema? An analysis of systematic reviews published in 2008 and 2009.*Clin. Exp. Dermatol.*2010;35:823-828.
[245] Joint Task Force on Practice Parameters; American Academy of Allergy, Asthma and Immunology; American College of Allergy, Asthma and Immunology; Joint Council of Allergy, Asthma and Immunology.The diagnosis and management of anaphylaxis: an updated practice parameter.*J. Allergy Clin. Immunol.*2005;115:S483-S523.
[246] Leung, AK; Leung, JS.Food allergy.New York: Nova Science Publishers, Inc., 2010, pp.1-83.
[247] Hon, KLE; Leung, TF; Kam, WYC; et al. Dietary restriction and supplementation in children with atopic eczema.*Clin. Exp. Dermatol.* 2006;31:187-191.
[248] Leung, AK; Hon, KL.Management of the child with food allergy.In: Chesterton, CM. (ed).*Food Allergies: New Research*.New York: Nova Science Publishers, Inc., 2008, pp.135-156.
[249] American Academy of Pediatrics.Food sensitivity.In:Kleinman, RE. (ed). *Pediatric Nutrition Handbook*. 6th ed. Elk Grove Village, IL: American Academy of Pediatrics, 2008, pp.783-799.
[250] Hanifin, JM; Cooper, KD; Ho, VC; et al.Guidelines of care for atopic dermatitis.*J. Am. Acad. Dermatol.* 2004;50:391-404.
[251] Muraro, A; Dreborg, S; Halken, S; et al.Dietary prevention of allergic diseases in infants and small children.Part III: critical review of published peer-reviewed observational and interventional studies and final recommendations.*Pediatr. Allergy Immunol.*2004;15:291-307.
[252] Yang, YW; Tsai, CL; Lu, CY.Exclusive breastfeeding and incident atopic dermatitis in childhood: a systematic review and meta-analysis of prospective cohort studies.*Br. J. Dermatol.*2009;161:373-383.
[253] Leung, AK; Sauve, RS.Breast is best for babies.*J. Natl. Med. Assoc.*2005;97:1010-1019.
[254] Brostoff, J; Hawk, LJ.Food allergy in children.*Eur. J. Nutr.*1991;45:S11-S15.

[255] Zeiger, RS. Prevention of food allergy in infancy. *Ann. Allergy.* 1990;65:430-441.
[256] Oddy, WH; Rosales, F. A systematic review of the importance of milk TGF-beta on immunological outcomes in the infant and young child. *Pediatr. Allergy Immunol.* 2009;21:47-59.
[257] Greer, FR; Siccherer, SH; Burks, AW; et al. Effects of early nutritional interventions on the development of atopic disease in infants and children: the role of maternal dietary restriction, breastfeeding, timing of introduction of complementary foods, and hydrolyzed formulas. *Pediatrics.* 2008;121:183-191.
[258] Simpson, EL. Atopic dermatitis prevention. *Dermatol. Ther.* 2006;19:108-117.
[259] Thygarajan, A; Burks, AW. American Academy of Pediatrics recommendations on the effects of early nutritional interventions on the development of atopic disease. *Curr. Opin. Pediatr.* 2008;20:698-702.
[260] Alexander, DD; Cabana, MD. Partially hydrolyzed 100% whey protein infant formula and reduced risk of atopic dermatitis: a meta-analysis. *J. Pediatr. Gastroenterol. Nutr.* 2010;50:422-430.
[261] Berg, A; Krämer, U; Link, E; et al. Impact of early feeding on childhood eczema: development after nutritional intervention compared with the natural course – the GINIplus study up to the age of 6 years. *Clin. Exp. Allergy.* 2010;40:627-636.
[262] von Berg, A; Koletzko, S; Grübl, A; et al. The effect of hydrolyzed cow's milk formula for allergy prevention in the first year of life: the German Infant Nutritional Intervention Study, a randomized double-blind trial. *J. Allergy Clin. Immunol.* 2003;111:533-540.
[263] Iskedjian, M; Szajewska, H; Spieldenner, J; et al. Meta-analysis of a partially hydrolysed 100%-whey infant formula vs. extensively hydrolysed infant formulas in the prevention of atopic dermatitis. *Curr. Med. Res. Opin.* 2010;26:2599-2606.
[264] Kramer, MS; Kakuma, R. Maternal dietary antigen avoidance during pregnancy or lactation, or both, for preventing or treating atopic disease in the child. *Cochrane Database Syst. Rev.* 2006;3:CD000133.
[265] Lynde, C; Barber, K; Claveau, J; et al. Canadian Practical Guide for the Treatment and Management of Atopic Dermatitis. *J. Cutan. Med. Surg.* http://www.springerlink.com/content/r5432000056r2748/ [last accessed on December 9, 2010].
[266] Simpson, EL. Atopic dermatitis: a review of topical treatment options. *Curr. Med. Res. Opin.* 2010;26:633-640.

[267] Lucky, AW; Leach, AD; Laskarzewski, P; et al. Use of an emollient as a steroid-sparing agent in the treatment of mild to moderate atopic dermatitis in children. *Pediatr. Dermatol.* 1997;14:321-324.
[268] Lancaster, W. Atopic eczema in infants and children: working with children and their families to manage eczema and control flare-ups. *Community Pract.* 2009;82:36-37.
[269] Bissonnette, R; Maari, C; Provost, N; et al. A double-blind study of tolerance and efficacy of a new urea-containing moisturizer in patients with atopic dermatitis. *J. Cosmet. Dermatol.* 2010;9:16-21.
[270] Chamlin, SL; Frieden, IJ; Fowler, A; et al. Ceramide-dominant, barrier-repair lipids improve childhood atopic dermatitis. *Arch. Dermatol.* 2001;137:1110-1112.
[271] Draelos, ZD. The effect of ceramide-containing skin care products on eczema resolution duration. *Cutis.* 2008;81:87-91.
[272] Ellias, PM; Wakefield, JS. Therapeutic implications of a barrier-based pathogenesis of atopic dermatitis. *Clin. Rev. Allergy Immunol.* (in press).
[273] Madaan, A. Epiceram for the treatment of atopic dermatitis. *Drugs Today.* 2008;44:751-755.
[274] Hon, KL; Wang, SS; Lau, Z; et al. Pseudoceramide for childhood eczema: does it work? *Hong Kong Med. J.* 2011;17:132-136.
[275] Patrizi, A; Capitanio, B; Neri, I; et al. A double-blind, randomized, vehicle-controlled clinical study to evaluate the efficacy and safety of MAS063DP (ATOPICLAIR^{TM}) in the management of atopic dermatitis in paediatric patients. *Pediatr. Allergy Immunol.* 2008;19:619-625.
[276] Hon, KL; Ching, GK; Leung, TF; et al. Estimating emollient usuage in patients with eczema. *Clin. Exp. Dermatol.* 2009;35:22-26.
[277] Gimalt, R; Mengeaud, V; Cambazard, F. The steroid-sparing effect of an emollient therapy in infants with atopic dermatitis: a randomized controlled study. *Dermatology.* 2007;214:61-67.
[278] Almawi, WY; Melemedjian, OK. Molecular mechanisms of glucocorticoid antiproliferative effects: antagonism of transcription factors activity by glucocorticoid receptor. *J. Leukoc. Biol.* 2002;71:9-15.
[279] Alomar, A; Berth-Jones, J; Bos, JD; et al. The role of topical calcineurin inhibitors in atopic dermatitis. *Br. J. Dermatol.* 2004;151(Suppl 70):3-27.
[280] Lebwohl, M. A comparison of once-daily application of mometasone furoate 0.1% cream compared with twice-daily hydrocortisone valerate 0.2% cream in pediatric atopic dermatitis patients who failed to respond to hydrocortisone: mometasone furoate study group. *Int. J. Dermatol.* 1999;38:604-606.

[281] Wolkerstorfer, A; Strobos, MA; Glazenburg, EJ; et al. Fluticasone propionate 0.05% cream once daily versus clobetasone butyrate 0.05% cream twice daily in children with atopic dermatitis. *J. Am. Acad. Dermatol.* 1998;39:226-231.
[282] Carr, JD. Evidence-based management of childhood atopic eczema. *Br. J. Nurs.* 2009;18:603-610.
[283] van Velsen, SG; Haeck, IM; Bruijnzeel-Koomen, CA. Percutaneous absorption of potent topical corticocorticoids in patients with severe atopic dermatitis. *J. Am. Acad. Dermatol.* 2010;63:911-913.
[284] Callen, J; Chamlin, S; Eichenfield, LF; et al. A systematic review of the safety of topical therapies for atopic dermatitis. *Br. J. Dermatol.* 2007;156:203-221.
[285] Langley, RG; Eichenfield, LF; Lucky, AW; et al. Sustained efficacy and safety of pimecrolimus cream 1% when used long-term (up to 26 weeks) to treat children with atopic dermatitis. *Pediatr. Dermatol.* 2008;25:301-307.
[286] Kondo, Y; Nakajima, Y; Komatsubara, R; et al. Short-term efficacy of tacrolimus ointment and impact on quality of life. *Pediatr. Int.* 2009;51:385-389.
[287] Kang, S; Lucky, AW; Pariser, D, et al. Long-term safety and efficacy of tacrolimus ointment for the treatment of atopic dermatitis in children. *J. Am. Acad. Dermatol.* 2001;44:S58-S64.
[288] Paller, AS; Eichenfield, LF; Kirsner, RS; et al. Three times weekly tacrolimus oitment reduces relapse in stabilized atopic dermatitis: a new paradigm for use. *Pediatrics.* 2008;122:e1210-e1218.
[289] Thaçi, D; Reitamo, S; Ensenat, G; et al. Proactive disease management with 0.03% tacrolimus ointment for children with atopic dermatitis: results of a randomized, multicentre, comparative study. *Br. J. Dermatol.* 2008;159:1348-1356.
[290] Kubota, Y; Yoneda, K; Nakai, K. Effect of sequential applications of topical tacrolimus and topical corticosteroids in the treatment of pediatric atopic dermatitis: an open-label pilot study. *J. Am. Acad. Dermatol.* 2009;60:212-217.
[291] Bekersky, I; Fitzsimmons, W; Tanase, A; et al. Nonclinical and early clinical development of tacrolimus ointment for the treatment of atopic dermatitis. *J. Am. Acad. Dermatol.* 2001;44:S17-S27.
[292] Reitamo, S; Rissanen, J; Remitz, A; et al.Tacrolimus ointment does not affect collagen synthesis: results of a single-center randomized trial.*J. Invest. Dermatol.*1998;111:396-398.

[293] Allen, BR.Tacrolimus ointment: its place in the therapy of atopic dermatitis.*J. Allergy Clin. Immunol.*2002;109:401-403.
[294] Hauk, PJ; Leung, DY.Tacrolimus (FK 506): new treatment approach in superantigen-associated diseases like atopic dermatitis?*J. Allergy Clin. Immunol.*2001;107:391-392.
[295] Eichenfield, LF; Thaci, D; de Prost, Y; et al.Clinical management of atopic eczema with pimecrolimus cream 1% (Elidel®) in paediatric patients.*Dermatology.*2007;215(Suppl 1):3-17.
[296] Arkwright, PD; Patel, L; Moran, A; et al.Atopic eczema is associated with delayed maturation of the antibody response to pneumococcal vaccine.*Clin. Exp. Immunol.* 2000;122:16-19.
[297] Stiehm, ER; Roberts, RL; Kaplan, MS; et al.Pneumococcal seroconversion after vaccination in children with atopic dermatitis treated with tacrolimus ointment.*J. Am. Acad. Dermatol.*2005;53:S206-S213.
[298] Bernard, LA; Eichenfield, LF.Topical immunomodulators for atopic dermatitis.*Curr. Opin. Pediatr.*2002;14:414-418.
[299] Wollenberg, A; Sharma, S; von Bubnoff, D; et al.Topical tacrolimus (FK506) leads to profound phenotypic and functional alterations of epidermal antigen-presenting dendritic cells in atopic dermatitis.*J. Allergy Clin. Immunol.* 2001;107:519-525.
[300] Caproni, M; Torchia, D; Antiga, E; et al. The effects of tacrolimus ointment on regulatory T lymphocytes in atopic dermatitis.*J. Clin. Immunol.*2006;26:370-375.
[301] Grassberger, M; Baumrucker, T; Enz, A; et al. A novel anti-inflammatory drug, SDZ ASM 981, for the treatment of skin diseases: *in vitro* pharmacology.*Br. J. Dermatol.* 1999;141:24-73.
[302] Hultsch, T; Muller, KD; Meingassner, JG; et al. Ascomycin macrolactam derivative SDZ ASM 981 inhibits the release of granule-associated mediators and of newly synthesized cytokines in RBL 2H3 mast cells in an immunophilin-dependent manner.*Arch. Dermatol. Res.*1998;290:501-507.
[303] Meingassner, JG; Grassberger, M; Fahrngruber, H; et al. A novel anti-inflammatory drug, SDZ ASM 981, for the topical and oral treatment of skin diseases: *in vivo* pharmacology.*Br. J. Dermatol.* 1997;137:568-576.
[304] Iskedjian, M; Piwko, C; Shear, NH; et al.Topical calcineurin inhibitors in the treatment of atopic dermatitis: a meta-analysis of current evidence.*Am. J. Clin. Dermatol.* 2004;5:267-279.
[305] Ashcroft, DM; Dimmock, P; Garside, R; et al. Efficacy and tolerability of topical pimecrolimus and tacrolimus in the treatment of atopic dermatitis: meta-analysis of randomised controlled trials.*BMJ.*2005;330:516.

[306] Bigby, M.Tacrolimus and pimecrolimus for atopic dermatitis: where do they fit in?*Arch. Dermatol.*2006;142:1203-1205.
[307] Kempers, S; Boguniewicz, M; Carter, E; et al.A randomized investigator-blinded study comparing pimecrolimus cream 1% with tacrolimus ointment 0.03% in the treatment of pediatric patients with moderate atopic dermatitis.*J. Am. Acad. Dermatol.* 2004;51:515-525.
[308] Paller, AS; Lebwohl, M; Fleischer, AB, Jr.; et al. Tacrolimus ointment is more effective than pimecrolimus cream with a similar safety profile in the treatment of atopic dermatitis: results from 3 randomized, comparative studies.*J. Am. Acad. Dermatol.* 2005;52:810-822.
[309] Yan, J; Chen, SL; Wang, XL; et al. Meta-analysis of tacrolimus ointment for atopic dermatitis in pediatric patients.*Pediatr. Dermatol.*2008;25:117-120.
[310] Chen, SL; Yan, J; Wang, FS.Two topical calcineurin inhibitors for the treatment of atopic dermatitis in pediatric patients: a meta-analysis of randomized clinical trials.*J. Dermatol. Treat.*2010;21:144-156.
[311] Kirsner, RS; Heffernan, MP; Antaya, R.Safety and efficacy of tacrolimus ointment versus pimecrolimus cream in the treatment of patients with atopic dermatitis previously treated with corticosteroids.*Acta Derm. Venereol.*2010;90:58-64.
[312] Doss, N; Kamoun, MR; Dubertret, L; et al.Efficacy of tacrolimus 0.03% ointment as second-line treatment for children with moderate-to-severe atopic dermatitis: evidence from a randomized, double-blind non-inferiority trial vs. fluticasone 0.005% ointment.*Pediatr. Allergy Immunol.*2010;21:321-329.
[313] Fonacier, L; Spergel, J; Charlesworth, EN; et al.Report of the Topical Calcineurin Task Force of the American College of Allergy, Asthma and Immunology and the American Academy of Allergy, Asthma and Immunology.*J. Allergy Clin. Immunol.*2005;115:1249-1253.
[314] Fonacier, L; Charlesworth, EN; Spergel, J; et al.The black box warning for topical calcineurin inhibitors: looking outside the box.*Ann. Allergy Asthma. Immunol.*2006;97:117-120.
[315] Carroll, CL; Fleischer, AB, Jr.Tacrolimus: focusing on atopic dermatitis.*Drugs Today.*2006;42:431-439.
[316] Akdis, CA; Akdi, M; Bieber, T; et al. Diagnosis and treatment of atopic dermatitis in children and adults: European Academy of Allergology and Clinical Immunology/American Academy of Allergy, Asthma and Immunology/PRACTALL Consensus Report. *Allergy.* 2006;61:969-987.

[317] Margolis, D; Hoffstad, O; Bilker, W. Lack of association between exposure to topical calcineurin inhibitors and skin cancers in adults. *Dermatology.* 2007;214:289-295.
[318] Thaçi, D; Salgo, R. Malignancy concerns of topical calcineurin inhibitors for atopic dermatitis: facts and controversies. *Clin. Dermatol.* 2010;28:52-56.
[319] Schmitt, J; Schmitt, N; Meurer, M. Cyclosporin in the treatment of patients with atopic eczema: a systematic review and meta-analysis. *J. Eur. Acad. Dermatol. Venereol.* 2007;21:606-619.
[320] Heller, M; Shin, HT; Orlow, SJ; et al. Mycophenolate mofetil for severe childhood atopic dermatitis: experience in 14 patients. *Br. J. Dermatol.* 2007;157:127-132.
[321] Leung, AK; Wong, BE; Chan, PY; et al. Pruritus in children. *J. R. Soc. Health.* 1998;118:280-286.
[322] Schnopp, C; Ring, J; Mempel, M. The role of antibacterial therapy in atopic dermatitis. *Expert Opin. Pharmacother.* 2010;11:929-936.
[323] Moody, MN; Morrison, LK; Tyring, SK; et al. Retapamulin: what is the role of this topical antimicrobial in the treatment of bacterial infections in topical dermatitis? *Skin Therapy Lett.* 2010;15:1-4.
[324] Free, A; Roth, E; Dalessandro, M; et al. Retapamulin ointment twice daily for 5 days vs oral cephalexin twice daily for 10 days for empiric treatment of secondarily infected traumatic lesions of the skin. *Skinmed.* 2006;5:224-232.
[325] Parish, LC; Jorizzo, JL; Breton, JJ; et al. Topical retapamulin oitment (1% wt/wt) twice daily for 5 days versus oral cephalexin twice daily for 10 days in the treatment of secondarily infected dermatitis: results of a randomized controlled trial. *J. Am. Acad. Dermatol.* 2006;55:1003-1013.
[326] Bath-Hextall, FJ; Birnie, AJ; Ravenscroft, JC; et al. Interventions to reduce *Staphylococcus aureus* in the management of atopic eczema: an updated Cochrane review. *Br. J. Dermatol.* 2010;163:12-26.
[327] Craig, FE; Smith, EV; Williams, HC; et al. Bleach baths to reduce severity of atopic dermatitis colonized by *Staphylococcus*. *Arch. Dermatol.* 2010;146:541-543.
[328] Tan, WP; Suresh, S; Tey, HL; et al. A randomized double-blind controlled trial to compare a triclosan-containing emollient with vehicle for the treatment of atopic dermatitis. *Clin Exp. Dermatol.* 2009;35:e109-e112.
[329] Stalder, JF; Fleury, M; Sourisse, M; et al. Comparative effects of two topical antiseptics (chlorhexidine vs KMnO4) on bacterial skin flora in atopic dermatitis. *Acta Derm. Venereol. Suppl. (Stockh)* 1992;176:132-134.

[330] Garvey, LH; Kroigaard, M; Poulsen; et al. IgE-mediated allergy to chlohexidine. *J. Allergy Clin. Immunol.* 2007;120:409-415.

[331] Jee, R; Nel, L; Gnanakumaran, G; et al. Four cases of anaphylaxis to chlorhexidine impregnated central venous catheters: a case cluster or the tip of the iceberg? *Br. J. Anaesth.* 2009;103:614-615.

[332] Gauger, A. Silver-coated textiles in the therapy of atopic eczema. *Curr. Probl. Dermatol.* 2006;33:152-164.

[333] Gauger, A; Fisher, S; Mempel, M; et al. Efficacy and functionality of silver-coated textiles in patients with atopic eczema. *J. Eur. Acad. Dermatol. Venereol.* 2006;18:534-541.

[334] Haug,S; Roll,A; Schmid-Grendelmeier,P; et al. Coated textiles in the treatment of atopic dermatitis. *Curr. Probl. Dermatol.* 2006;33:144-151.

[335] Juenger,M; Ladwig,A; Staecker,S; et al. Efficacy and safety of silver textile in the treatment of atopic dermatitis (AD). *Curr. Med. Res. Opin.* 2006; 22:739-750.

[336] Ricci, G; Patrizi, A; Bellini, F; et al. Use of textiles in atopic dermatitis. *Curr. Probl. Dermatol.* 2006;33:127-143.

[337] Koller, DY; Halmerbauer, G; Böck, A. Action of a silk fabric treated with AEGIS™ in children with atopic dermatitis: a 3-month trial. *Pediatr. Allergy Immunol.* 2007;18:335-338.

[338] Senti, G; Steinmann, LS; Fischer, B; et al. Antimicrobial silk clothing in the treatment of atopic dermatitis proves comparable to topical corticosteroid treatment. *Dermatology.* 2006;213:228-233.

[339] Clayton, TH; Clark, SM; Turner, D; et al. The treatment of severe atopic dermatitis in childhood with narrowband ultraviolet B phototherapy. *Clin. Exp. Dermatol.* 2006;32:28-33.

[340] Sezer, E; Etikan, I. Local narrowband UVB phototherapy vs. local PUVA in the treatment of chronic hand eczema. *Photodermatol. Photoimmunol. Photomed.* 2007;23:10-14.

[341] Barham, KL; Yosipovitch, G. It's a wrap: the use of wet pajamas in wet-wrap dressings for atopic dermatitis. *Dermatol. Nurs.* 2005;17: 365-367.

[342] Devillers, ACA; Oranje, AP. Efficacy and safety of 'wet-wrap' dressings as an intervention treatment in children with severe and/or refractory atopic dermatitis: a critical review of the literature. *Br. J. Dermatol.* 2006;154:579-585.

[343] Hon, KL; Wong, KY; Cheung, LK; et al. Efficacy and problems associated with using a wet-wrap garment for children with severe atopic dermatitis. *J. Dermatol. Treat.* 2007;18:301-305.

[344] Bingham, LG; Noble, JW; Davis, MD. Wet dressings used with topical corticosteroids for pruritic dermatosis: a retrospective study. *J. Am. Acad. Dermatol.* 2009;60:792-800.

[345] National Patient Safety Agency. Fire hazard with paraffin-based skin products on dressings and clothing. www.npsa.nhs.uk/patient-safety-videos/parffib-based-skin-products/ [last accessed on December 9, 2010].

[346] Hessle, C; Hanson, LÅ; Wold, AE. Lactobacilli from human gastrointestinal mucosa are strong stimulators of IL-12 production. *Clin. Exp. Immunol.* 1999;116:276-282.

[347] Kirjavainen, PV; Apostolou, E; Salminen, SJ; et al. New aspects of probiotics – a novel approach in the management of food allergy. *Allergy.* 1999;54:909-915.

[348] Paganelli, R; Ciuffreda, S; Verna, N; et al. Probiotics and food-allergic diseases. *Allergy.* 2002;57:97-99.

[349] Williams, HC; Grindlay, DJ. What's new in atopic dermatitis? An analysis of systematic reviews published in 2007 and 2008. Part 2. Disease prevention and treatment. *Clin. Exp. Dermatol.* 2009;35:223-227.

[350] Williams, HC. Two "positive" studies of probiotics for atopic dermatitis – or are they? *Arch. Dermatol.* 2006;142:1201-1203.

[351] Kalliomäki, M; Salminen, S; Arvilommi, H; et al. Probiotics in primary prevention of atopic disease: a randomised placebo-controlled trial. *Lancet.* 2001;357:1076-1079.

[352] Kalliomäki, M; Isolauri, E. Role of intestinal flora in the development of allergy. *Curr. Opin. Allergy Clin. Immunol.* 2003;3:15-20.

[353] Lodinová-Zádníková,R; Cukrowska,B; Tlaskalova-Hogenova,H. Oral administration of probiotic *Escherichia coli* after birth reduces frequency of allergies and repeated infections later in life (after 10 and 20 years). *Int. Arch. Allergy Immunol.* 2003;131:209-211.

[354] Rosenfeldt, V; Benfeldt, E; Nielsen, SD; et al. Effect of probiotic *lactobacillus* strains in children with atopic dermatitis. *J. Allergy Clin. Immunol.* 2003;111:389-395.

[355] Soh, SE; Gerez, I; Chong, YS; et al. Probiotic supplementation in the first 6 months of life in at risk Asian infants – effects on eczema on atopic sensitization at the age of 1 year. *Clin. Exp. Allergy.* 2009;39:571-578.

[356] Viljanen,M; Savilahti,E; Haahtela, T; et al. Probiotics in the treatment of atopic eczema/dermatitis syndrome in infants: a double-blind placebo-controlled trial. *Allergy.* 2005;60:494-500.

[357] Weston, S; Halbert, A; Richmond, P; et al. Effects of probiotics on atopic dermatitis: a randomised controlled trial. *Arch. Dis. Child.* 2005;90:892-897.

[358] Boyle, RJ; Ismail, IH; Kivivuori, S; et al. *Lactobacillus* GG treatment during pregnancy for the prevention of eczema: a randomized controlled trial. *Allergy.* 2010;doi:10.1111/j.1398-9995.2010.02507.x

[359] Niers, L; Martin, R; Rijkers, G; et al. The effects of selected probiotic strains on the development of eczema (the PandA study). *Allergy.* 2009;64:1349-1358.

[360] Passeron,T; Lacour,JP; Fontas, E; et al. Prebiotics and synbiotics: two promising approaches for the treatment of atopic dermatitis in children above 2 years.*Allergy.*2006;61:431-437.

[361] van der Aa, LB; Heymans, HS; van Aalderen, WM; et al. Effect of a new synbiotic mixture on atopic dermatitis in infants: a randomized-controlled trial. *Clin. Exp. Allergy.* 2010;40:795-804.

[362] Boyle, RJ; Bath-Hextall, FJ; Leonardi-Bee, J; et al.Probiotics for treating eczema.*Cochrane Database Syst. Rev.*2008;4:CD006135.

[363] Lee, J; Seto, D; Bielory, L.Meta-analysis of clinical trials of probiotics for prevention and treatment of pediatric atopic dermatitis.*J. Allergy Clin. Immunol.* 2008;121:116-121.

[364] Fölster-Holst, R.Probiotics in the treatment and prevention of atopic dermatitis.*Ann. Nutr. Metab.*2010;57(Suppl):16-19.

[365] Lee, J; Bielory, L.Complementary and alternative interventions in atopic dermatitis.*Immunol. Allergy Clin. North Am.*2010;30:411-424.

[366] van der Aa, LB; Heymans, HS; van Aalderen, WM; et al. Probiotics and prebiotics in atopic dermatitis: review of the theoretical background and clinical evidence. *Pediatr. Allergy Immunol.* 2010;21:e355-e367.

[367] Broshtilova, V; Gantcheva, M.Cysteinyl leukotriene receptor antagonist montelukast in the treatment of atopic dermatitis.*Dermatol. Ther.*2010;23:90-93.

[368] Capella, GL; Grigerio, E; Altomare, G.A randomized trial of leukotriene receptor antagonist montelukast in moderate-to-severe atopic dermatitis of adults.*Eur. J. Dermatol.* 2001;11:209-213.

[369] Ehlayel, MS; Bener, A; Sabbah, A.Montelukast treatment in children with moderately severe atopic dermatitis.*Eur. Ann. Allergy Clin. Immunol.* 2007;39:232-236.

[370] Friedmann, PS; Palmer, R; Tan, E.A double-blind, placebo-controlled trial of montelukast in adult.*Clin. Exp. Allergy.*2007;37:1536-1540.

[371] Hon, KLE; Leung, TF; Ma, KC; et al. Brief case series: montelukast, at doses recommended for asthma treatment, reduces disease severity and increases soluble CD14 in children with atopic dermatitis.*J. Dermatol. Treat.*2005;16:15-18.
[372] Pei, AYS; Chan, HHL; Leung, TF.Montelukast in the treatment of children with moderate-to-severe atopic dermatitis: a pilot study.*Pediatr. Allergy Immunol.*2001;12:154-158.
[373] Yanase, DJ; David-Bajar, K.The leukotriene antagonist montelukast as a therapeutic agent for atopic dermatitis.*J. Am. Acad. Dermatol.*2001;44:89-93.
[374] Bussmann, C; Maintz, L; Hart, J; et al.Clinical improvement and immunological changes in atopic dermatitis patients undergoing subcutaneous immunotherapy with a house dust mite allergoid: a pilot study.*Clin. Exp. Allergy.*2007;37:1277-1285.
[375] Czarnecka-Operacz, M; Silny, W.Specific immunotherapy in atopic dermatitis.*Acta Dermatovenerol. Croat.*2006;14:52-59.
[376] Pajno, GB; Caminiti, L; Vita, D; et al. Sublingual immunotherapy in mite-sensitized children with atopic dermatitis: a randomized, double-blind, placebo-controlled study. *J. Allergy Clin. Immunol.* 2007;120:164-170.
[377] Werfel, T; Breuer, K; Rueff, F; et al. Usefulness of specific immunotherapy in patients with atopic dermatitis and allergic sensitization to house dust mites: a multi-centre, randomized, dose-response study.*Allergy.* 2006;61:202-205.
[378] Cadario, G; Galluccio, AG; Pezza, M; et al.Sublingual immunotherapy efficacy in patients with atopic dermatitis and house dust mites sensitivity: a prospective pilot study.*Curr. Med. Res. Opin.*2007;23:2503-2506.
[379] Glover, MT; Atherton, DJ.A double-blind controlled trial of hyposensitization to *Dermatophagoides pteronyssinus* in children with atopic eczema.*Clin. Exp. Allergy.* 1992;22:440-446.
[380] Mastrandrea, F.The potential role of allergen-specific sublingual immunotherapy in atopic dermatitis.*Am. J. Clin. Dermatol.*2004;5:281-294.
[381] Hughes, R; Ward, D; Tobin, AM; et al. The use of alternative medicine in pediatric patients with atopic dermatitis.*Pediatr. Dermatol.*2007;24:118-120.
[382] Hon, KLE; Leung, TF; Wong, Y; et al.A pentaherbs capsule as a treatment option for atopic dermatitis in children: an open-labeled case series.*Am. J. Clin. Med.* 2004;32:941-950.
[383] Hon, KL; Leung, TF; Ng, PC; et al. Efficacy and tolerability of a Chinese herbal medicine concoction for treatment of atopic dermatitis: a

randomized, double-blind, placebo-controlled study. *Br. J. Dermatol.* 2007;157:357-363.

[384] Sheehan, MP; Atherton, DJ. One-year follow up of children treated with Chinese medicinal herbs for atopic eczema. *Br. J. Dermatol.* 1994;130:488-493.

[385] Hon, KL; Leung, AK. Powerful proprietary Chinese medicine for eczema? *Clin. Exp. Dermatol.* 2010;35:e14-e15.

[386] Kang, KD; Kang, SM; Yim, HB. Herbal medication aggravates cataract formation: a case report. *J. Korean Med. Sci.* 2008;23:537-539.

[387] Ramsay, HM; Goddard, W; Gill, S; et al. Herbal creams used for atopic eczema in Birmingham, UK illegally contain potent corticosteroids. *Arch. Dis. Child.* 2003; 88:1056-1057.

[388] Bukutu, C; Deol, J; Shamseer, L; et al. Complementary, holistic, and integrative medicine: atopic dermatitis. *Pediatr. Rev.* 2007;28:e87-e94.

[389] Ferguson,JE; Chalmers, RJ; Rowlands, DJ. Reversible dilated cardiomyopathy following treatment of atopic eczema with Chinese herbal medicine. *Br. J. Dermatol.* 1997;136:592-593.

[390] Perharic, L; Shaw, D; Leon, C; et al. Possible association of liver damage with the use of Chinese herbal medicine for skin disease. *Vet. Human Toxicol.* 1995;37:562-566.

[391] Hon, KL; Lo, W; Cheng, WK; et al. Prospective self-controlled trial of the efficacy and tolerability of a herbal syrup for young children with eczema. *J. Dermatol. Treat.* (In press).

[392] Hon, KL; Lee, VW; Leung, TF; et al. Corticosteroids are not present in a traditional Chinese medicine formulation for atopic dermatitis in children. *Ann. Acad. Med. Singapore.* 2006;35:759-763.

[393] Lee, J; Jung, E; Koh, J; et al. Effect of rosmarinic acid on atopic dermatitis. *J. Dermatol.* 2008;35:768-771.

[394] Senapati, S; Banerjee, S; Gangopadhyay, DN. Evening primrose oil is effective in atopic dermatitis: a randomized placebo-controlled trial. *Indain J. Dermatol. Venereol.* 2008;74:447-452.

[395] Anandan, C; Nurmatov, U; Sheikh, A. Omega 3 and 6 oils for primary prevention of allergic disease: systematic review and meta-analysis. *Allergy.* 2009;64:840-848.

[396] Hoppu, U; Rinne, M; Lampi, AM; et al. Breast milk fatty acid composition is associated with development of atopic dermatitis in the infant. *J. Pediatr. Gastroenterol. Nutr.* 2005;41:335-338.

[397] Dunstan, JA; Mori, TA; Barden, A; et al. Fish oil supplementation in pregnancy reduces interleukin-13 levels in cord blood of infants at high risk of atopy. *Clin. Exp. Allergy.* 2002;33:442-448.
[398] Dunstan, JA; Mori, TA; Barden, A; et al. Fish oil supplementation in pregnancy modifies neonatal allergen-specific immune responses and clinical outcomes in infants at high risk of atopy: a randomized, controlled trial. *J. Allergy Clin. Immunol.* 2003;112:1178-1184.
[399] Kitz, R; Rose, MA; Schonborn, H; et al. Impact of early dietary gamma-linoleic acid supplementation on atopic eczema in infancy. *Pediatr. Allergy Immunol.* 2006;17:112-117.
[400] Rasmussen, JE. Advances in nondietary management of children with atopic dermatitis. *Pediatr. Dermatol.* 1989;6:210-215.
[401] Takwale, A; Tan, E; Agarwal, S; et al. Efficacy and tolerability of borage oil in adults and children with atopic eczema: randomised, double blind, placebo controlled, parallel group trial. *BMJ.* 2003;13:1385.
[402] van Gool, CJ; Zeegers, MP; Thijs, C. Oral essential acid supplementation in atopic dermatitis – a meta-analysis of placebo-controlled trials. *Br. J. Dermatol.* 2004;150:728-740.
[403] Morse, NL; Clough, PM. A meta-analysis of randomized, placebo-controlled clinical trials of Efamol® evening primrose oil in atopic eczema. Where do we go from here in light of more recent discoveries? *Curr. Pharm. Biotechnol.* 2006;7:503-524.
[404] Foster, RH; Hardy, G; Alany, RG; et al. Borage oil in the treatment of atopic dermatitis. *Nutrition.* 2010;26:708-718.
[405] Solvoll, K; Søyland, E; Sandstad, B; et al. Dietary habits among patients with atopic dermatitis. *Eur. J. Clin. Nutr.* 2000;54:93-97.
[406] Bäck, O; Blomquist, HK; Hernell, O; et al. Does vitamin D intake during infancy promote the development of atopic allergy? *Acta Derm. Venereol.* 2009;89:28-32.
[407] Tsoureli-Nikita, E; Hercogova, J; Lotti, T; et al. Evaluation of dietary intake of vitamin E in the treatment of atopic dermatitis: a study of the clinical course and evaluation of the immunoglobulin E serum levels. *Int. J. Dermatol.* 2002;41:146-150.
[408] Javanbakht, MH; Keshavarz, SA; Djalali, M; et al. Randomized controlled trial using vitamins E and D supplementation in atopic dermatitis. *J. Dermatol. Treat.* (in press).
[409] Stücker, M; Pieck, C; Stoerb, C; et al. Topical vitamin B12 – a new therapeutic approach in atopic dermatitis – evaluation of efficacy and

tolerability in a randomized placebo-controlled multicentre clinical trial. *Br. J. Dermatol.* 2004;150:977-983.

[410] Kotani, M; Matsumoto, M; Fujita, A; et al. Persimmon leaf extract and astragalin inhibit development of dermatitis and IgE elevation in NC/Nga mice. *J. Allergy Clin. Immunol.* 2000;106:159-166.

[411] Matsumoto, M; Kotani, M; Fujita, A; et al. Oral administration of persimmon leaf extract ameliorates skin symptoms and transepidermal water loss in atopic dermatitis model mice, NC/Nga. *Br. J. Dermatol.* 2002;146:221-227.

[412] Tanaka, T; Kouda, K; Kotani, M; et al. Vegetarian diet ameliorates symptoms of atopic dermatitis through reduction of the number of peripheral eosinophils and of PGE2 synthesis by monocytes. *J. Physiol. Anthropol.* 2001;20:353-361.

[413] Beattie, PE; Lewis-Jones, MS. Parental knowledge of topical therapies in the treatment of childhood atopic dermatitis. *Clin. Exp. Dermatol.* 2003;28:549-553.

[414] Hon, KLE; Kam, WYC; Leung, TF; et al. Steroid fears in children with eczema. *Acta Paediatr.* 2006d;95:1451-1455.

[415] Hon, KL; Lee, VWY; Leung, TF; et al. Corticosteroids are not present in a traditional Chinese medicine formulation for atopic dermatitis in children.*Ann. Acad. Med. Singapore*.2006e;35:759-763.

[416] Zuberbier, T; Orlow, SJ; Paller, AS; et al. Patient perspectives on the management of atopic dermatitis. *J. Allergy Clin. Immunol.* 2006;118:226-232.

[417] Staab, D; Diepgen, TL; Fartasch, M; et al. Age related, structured educational programmes for the management of atopic dermatitis in children and adolescents: multicentre, randomised controlled trial. *BMJ.* 2006;332:933-936.

[418] Williams, HC. Atopic dermatitis. *N. Engl. J. Med.* 2005;352:2314-2324.

Index

A

accelerometers, 30
access, 43
acid, 10, 52, 62, 74, 75, 76, 77, 93, 118, 119
acne, 53
adhesion, 6, 8
adipose tissue, 53
adjustment, 103, 104
adolescents, viii, 19, 97, 120
adulthood, 95
adults, viii, ix, 3, 21, 26, 33, 52, 53, 54, 55, 57, 59, 73, 78, 92, 97, 106, 112, 116, 119
adverse effects, 53, 54, 61, 67, 73
adverse event, 55, 56, 57, 58
age, vii, ix, 8, 11, 13, 14, 19, 21, 23, 25, 26, 28, 31, 34, 35, 37, 42, 47, 51, 55, 60, 65, 67, 69, 72, 73, 74, 75, 79, 81, 87, 89, 98, 101, 108, 115
aggregation, 87
agonist, 10
agranulocytosis, 73
alanine, 71
alanine aminotransferase, 71
alkalinity, 9
allergens, vii, 1, 7, 8, 12, 21, 23, 38, 42, 45, 46, 50, 51, 94
allergic reaction, 62
allergic rhinitis, ix, 1, 31, 41, 81, 95
allergic sensitisation, 88
allergy, 12, 13, 42, 43, 46, 49, 62, 63, 69, 72, 88, 89, 94, 95, 105, 106, 107, 108, 113, 115, 119
alopecia, 33
alternative medicine, 73, 117
alters, 52
amino acid, 7
anaphylactic reactions, 64
anaphylaxis, 42, 95, 107, 113
animal dander, 14
antagonism, 109
antibiotic, 11, 62, 63, 102
antibody, 31, 42, 105, 111
anticholinergic, 62
anticholinergic effect, 62
antigen, 9, 12, 15, 31, 42, 47, 92, 108, 111
antihistamines, 45, 62, 64
antioxidant, 52
apoptosis, 6, 9, 12, 92
arsenic, 73
arthralgia, 61
aseptic, 60
ASI, 100
assessment, viii, 29, 32, 58, 59, 66, 100, 101, 102
asthma, ix, 1, 13, 20, 25, 31, 41, 72, 81, 86, 89, 95, 96, 100, 104, 116
asymptomatic, 33
Atopic dermatitis, vii, viii, 1, 3, 6, 15, 21, 36, 37, 38, 61, 81, 85, 86, 87, 88, 90, 95, 96,

97, 98, 99, 102, 103, 104, 105, 106, 108, 120
atopic eczema, 85, 87, 93, 94, 101, 103, 106, 107, 109, 110, 112, 113, 114, 115, 117, 118, 119
atopy, 3, 13, 15, 23, 26, 31, 42, 48, 87, 101, 106, 118
atrophy, 53, 54
avoidance, 14, 45, 46, 47, 50, 79, 108

B

bacteria, 8, 51, 69
bacterial infection, viii, 9, 35, 36, 62, 63, 113
bacterial strains, 68
bacterium, 11
basophils, 10, 93
baths, 51, 63, 64, 113
bedding, 46
beef, 13
Belgium, 87
beneficial effect, 10, 68, 76, 78
benefits, 59
birth weight, 50
blepharitis, 36
blood, 14, 118
body mass index, 3
bone, 60
bowel, 12
brain, 11, 94
breast milk, 48, 49, 75
breastfeeding, 47, 48, 49, 50, 107
bullying, 38

C

cadmium, 14
calcitonin, 15
calcitonin gene related peptide (CGRP), 15
cancer, 59
CAP, 72
capsule, 117
carbon dioxide, 100
carcinogenesis, 67
cardiomyopathy, 73
caregivers, 2, 38, 45, 47, 54, 78, 83
casein, 49, 50
cataract, 21, 73, 118
causal relationship, 60
causation, 48
cell death, 90
cell line, 52
cell lines, 52
central nervous system, 62
challenges, 12, 105
cheilitis, 22
chemicals, 7
chemokines, 16, 31
childhood, 2, 33, 38, 55, 81, 85, 86, 87, 89, 94, 96, 100, 101, 102, 103, 104, 105, 107, 108, 109, 113, 114, 120
Childhood Atopic Dermatitis Scale (CADIS), 31
China, ix, 73
Chinese medicine, 73, 117, 118, 120
chlorine, 46
cholesterol, 51
chromosome, 6, 88, 89
circulation, 15
classes, 3
classification, 39
climate, 46, 106
clinical symptoms, 10
clinical trials, viii, 32, 65, 76, 77, 112, 116, 119
Clinical validation, 99
clothing, 46, 64, 68, 114
coal, 66
coal tar, 66
cognitive function, 62
collagen, 54, 110
colonization, 9, 35, 55, 63, 64, 91, 93, 102
color, 35, 66
community, 35
complete blood count, 74
complex interactions, vii, 5
compliance, 47, 54, 78
complications, 36
composition, 7, 118
concordance, 5

conference, 28, 99
conjunctivitis, 26, 36
consensus, 48, 50, 99, 106
consumption, 65, 74
contact dermatitis, 33, 34, 66, 97
control group, 75
controlled studies, 50, 66, 73, 76
controlled trials, 47, 56, 58, 68, 70, 71, 73, 76, 78, 111, 119
controversial, 68, 77
controversies, 106, 112
cooling, 68
copper, 14
correlation, 3, 15, 46, 77, 86, 90, 103
corticosteroid cream, 64
corticosteroid therapy, 36
corticosteroids, ix, 36, 45, 52, 53, 54, 55, 56, 58, 60, 61, 64, 72, 73, 74, 79, 92, 110, 112, 114, 118
cost, 42, 67
cotton, 46, 64, 65
covering, 32, 65
Cox regression, 49
cracks, 21
cross-sectional study, 35
crust, 19, 29
culture, 10, 35
cure, 2, 79
curriculum, 37
cyclosporine, 43, 55, 61
cytokines, 6, 10, 16, 48, 52, 67, 68, 111
cytoskeleton, 7

D

defects, vii, 5, 7, 88, 89
deficiencies, 47
deficiency, 8, 75, 90
degradation, 7
dendritic cell, 10, 111
dermatologist, 6, 14, 35
dermatosis, vii, 1, 114
dermis, 17
detection, 10, 42
detergents, 45

developed countries, 3, 11
developing countries, 3
diabetes, 39
diagnostic criteria, 98, 99
diarrhea, 33
diet, 15, 47, 50, 78, 119, 120
differential diagnosis, 33, 102
dilated cardiomyopathy, 118
diphenhydramine, 62
discomfort, 61
disease activity, 11
diseases, 47, 87, 107, 110, 115
disorder, 3, 34, 85
dissatisfaction, 73
distress, 39
distribution, 26
dizygotic, 5
dizygotic twins, 5
dosage, 71, 74
dosing, 74
double-blind trial, 63, 108
down-regulation, 7
dressings, 46, 67, 114
drugs, 56, 60, 95

E

eczema, 1, 13, 25, 26, 34, 36, 52, 85, 86, 87, 89, 90, 93, 95, 96, 100, 101, 102, 104, 106, 108, 109, 111, 114, 115, 116, 117, 118, 120
Eczema Area and Severity Index (EASI), viii, 10, 29
edema, 17, 29, 30, 76
education, 45, 78
egg, 13, 46, 50
elbows, 33, 34
electrophoresis, 91
emergency, 43, 65
emotion, 31
encephalitis, 36
encephalopathy, 36, 103
endothelial cells, 6
energy, 100
energy expenditure, 100
England, 89

environment, 3, 46, 106
environmental factors, vii, 5, 23
environmental tobacco, 14, 96
eosinophil count, 13, 15, 74
eosinophilia, 2, 7, 9, 12, 17, 67, 120
epidemiology, 94
epidermis, 7, 17, 52
epithelial cells, 12, 91
epithelium, 21
equipment, 43
erythematous papules, viii, 21
essential fatty acids, 76, 77
Europe, 3
evaporation, 51, 67
evidence, vii, 1, 8, 11, 15, 47, 48, 49, 54, 63, 70, 73, 74, 106, 111, 112, 116
exclusion, 47, 71
exotoxins, 9, 92
exposure, 11, 12, 34, 36, 45, 46, 94, 112
extensor, vii, 19, 21, 25, 26, 34
extracellular matrix, 9
extracts, 42, 72

F

failure to thrive, 12, 34, 47
families, ix, 2, 3, 39, 70, 83, 101, 103, 108
family history, 13, 23, 26, 28, 48, 49, 69, 81
family members, 34, 54, 87
family studies, 6
fatty acids, 48, 51, 75, 76, 77
fear, 53, 73, 79, 120
fever, 13, 87
fibrinogen, 9, 91
fibroblasts, 55, 56
financial, 39, 83
fire hazard, 68
fish, 46, 76
flame, 68
flavonoids, 78
flaws, 47
flexor, 21
flora, 113
fluctuations, 37
fluid, 10

folliculitis, 35, 53, 66, 68
food, 1, 12, 13, 14, 39, 42, 43, 46, 47, 50, 68, 72, 75, 94, 95, 105, 107, 115
formation, 64, 73, 118
formula, 48, 49, 50, 70, 108
friction, 89
friendship, 38
fruits, 13
fungal infection, 36
fungi, 8, 93, 55

G

gastrointestinal tract, 68
gel, 91
genes, vii, 5, 52, 88
genetic predisposition, 5
genetics, 87, 88
genome, 88
gingival, 61
glaucoma, 53, 60
glomerulonephritis, 36
glossitis, 34
glucocorticoid receptor, 52, 55, 109
grading, 30, 100
granules, 7
growth, 34, 46, 53, 60, 68
guidelines, 43, 60, 99
guilt, 39

H

hay fever, 25
healing, 65
health, 43, 59, 68, 102, 104
heavy metals, 12, 14, 73, 96
helplessness, 39
hepatosplenomegaly, 34
herbal medicine, 73, 117, 118
herpes, viii, 36
herpes simplex, viii, 36
heterogeneity, 70
histamine, 6, 19, 61, 98
history, 1, 20, 25, 28, 41, 42, 48, 49, 69
Hong Kong, ix, 6, 109

host, 8, 68
house dust, 14, 46, 72, 96, 117
human, 11, 59, 78, 93, 115
humidity, 46
hydrocortisone, 55, 56, 58, 109
hygiene, 3
hyperesthesia, 61
hyperplasia, 17, 61
hypersensitivity, 12, 14, 37, 42, 47, 60, 95, 103, 105, 106
hypertension, 60, 61
hypertrichosis, 61

I

IFN, 61
IL-17, 31
immune response, 9, 54, 118
immune system, 11
immunity, 6, 26
immunization, 55
immunodeficiency, 33, 34
immunoglobulin, 92, 119
immunomodulation, 15
immunomodulator, 55
immunomodulatory, 74
immunosuppression, 60
immunotherapy, 72, 117
improvements, 58, 73
in utero, 50
in vitro, 111
in vivo, 111
incidence, 3, 21, 47, 48, 49, 57, 59, 69, 76, 94
income, 39
independence, 32
individuals, 10, 11, 12, 36, 41, 47, 55, 56, 72, 90
induction, 14
induration, 30
industrialization, vii, 1
ineffectiveness, 62
infancy, 2, 3, 33, 34, 86, 95, 107, 119
infants, vii, 8, 13, 19, 26, 43, 48, 49, 50, 51, 58, 68, 70, 75, 98, 100, 105, 107, 108, 109, 115, 116, 118

infection, 11, 35, 36, 46, 102
inferiority, 59, 112
inflammation, 6, 8, 9, 54
inflammatory cells, 6
inflammatory mediators, 6, 37
ingestion, 12
ingredients, 68
inhibition, 9, 67, 92
initiation, 10
injury, 46
insects, 96
insulin, 39
integrity, 51, 52, 53
interference, 42
interferon, 6, 61, 67
interferon gamma, 61
interferon-γ, 7, 67
internalization, 10
intervention, 49, 50, 69, 75, 76, 85, 108, 114
intestinal flora, 68, 115
irritability, 34, 37
issues, 31, 38

J

Japan, 51, 55, 102

K

keratin, 7
keratinocyte, 7, 8
keratinocytes, 8, 9, 16, 55, 56, 67
keratoconjunctivitis, 36, 103
keratosis, 21, 23, 26
knees, 33, 34

L

labeling, 60
lack of control, 47
lactation, 108
lactic acid, 74
lactobacillus, 115
Langerhans cells, 17, 55, 56, 67, 97

lead, 14, 45, 50, 53, 60, 96
legs, 66
lesions, viii, ix, 7, 9, 14, 15, 17, 21, 22, 28, 33, 34, 37, 43, 50, 52, 59, 62, 78, 93, 113
leukotrienes, 71
lichen, 22
life quality, 31
light, 19, 119
linoleic acid, 76, 119
lipids, 90, 109
liver, 118
liver damage, 118
localization, 8, 31, 34
loci, 5
loss of appetite, 37
lymph, 34
lymphadenopathy, 34
lymphocytes, 6, 15, 97
lymphoma, 59

M

macrophages, 9, 17
majority, 47
malignancy, 59, 61
malnutrition, 47
management, 12, 51, 78, 86, 91, 95, 96, 105, 107, 109, 110, 113, 115, 119, 120
marketing, 59
mass, 87
mast cells, 17, 19, 55, 56, 111
materials, 64
matrix, 7, 9
matter, viii, 29
measurement, viii, 14, 30, 31, 42, 103
measurements, 41
median, 59, 66
medical care, vii, 1
medication, 10, 38, 53, 55, 61, 65, 79, 118
medicine, 73, 74, 118
MEK, 93
melatonin, 11, 94
mellitus, 39
memory, 6, 31, 101
meningitis, 36

menstruation, 87
mercury, 14, 73
meta-analysis, 6, 49, 50, 56, 58, 61, 63, 70, 75, 76, 89, 107, 108, 111, 112, 118, 119
metals, 14
methodology, 48
mice, 15, 78, 119, 120
microorganisms, 11, 21, 68, 92
mitogen, 93
models, 70
modifications, 3
molds, 14
molecules, 6, 8, 9, 12, 42, 97
molluscum contagiosum, 36
monozygotic twins, 5
montelukast, 71, 116, 117
morphology, 26, 28
mucosa, 115
mutation, 8
mutations, 5, 7, 88, 89
myalgia, 61
myopathy, 60

N

nares, 9, 35, 63, 91
National Survey, 86
natural killer cell, 54
nausea, 61
necrosis, 60
neonates, 77
nervous system, 11
neuropeptides, 15, 31, 97
neutral, 45
neutrophils, 15, 17
nodules, 34
normal children, 39
Norway, 86
Nottingham Eczema Severity Score (NESS), viii, 14, 29
nuclear receptors, 11
nucleus, 52
null, 6, 88, 89
nummular eczema, 33, 34
nutrition, 49, 96

O

obesity, 60, 87
objectivity, 30, 43
occlusion, 16, 53, 97
oil, 51, 76, 77, 118, 119
oligosaccharide, 70
omega-3, 75, 76, 77
organism, 9
osteoporosis, 53, 60
outpatients, 64
oxygen consumption, 100

P

paediatric patients, 109, 110
pallor, 26, 28
papulovesicles, viii, 21
parallel, 119
parents, viii, 3, 15, 31, 32, 38, 49, 65, 91, 101, 102, 104
participants, 32, 56
pathogenesis, vii, 5, 7, 11, 71, 77, 83, 86, 89, 95, 97, 109
pathophysiology, 19
pathways, 6
PCR, 93
peptides, 8, 9, 15, 91
perinatal, 69
permeability, 5, 7, 8
personal history, 25
pH, 9, 45, 90
pharmacology, 111
pharmacotherapy, 2, 45, 79
phenotype, 89
phenotypes, 88
Philadelphia, 35, 95, 98
phobia, 53, 79
physicians, 59, 63
pigmentation, 67
pilot study, 105, 110, 116, 117
placebo, 12, 43, 47, 56, 64, 66, 68, 70, 72, 74, 75, 76, 77, 78, 94, 105, 115, 116, 117, 118, 119
plants, 46
playing, 46
PM, 92, 109, 119
pollution, vii, 1, 14
polymorphisms, 89
polythene, 16
polyunsaturated fat, 75, 76
polyunsaturated fatty acids, 75, 76
pools, 46
popliteal fossae, viii, 19
population, 86, 88, 94
positive correlation, viii, 31, 55
potassium, 64
pranlukast, 71
predictive accuracy, 42
pregnancy, 4, 50, 87, 108, 115, 118
preparation, 39, 66, 69, 72, 78
preschool, 86
preschool children, 86
prevention, 11, 50, 51, 68, 70, 75, 94, 105, 106, 107, 108, 115, 116, 118
probiotic, 69, 70, 115, 116
professionals, 43
pro-inflammatory, 67
proliferation, 6, 55
prophylactic, 75
protective mechanisms, 77
proteins, 5, 7, 8, 9, 91
pruritus, vii, ix, 1, 2, 6, 15, 19, 29, 37, 51, 59, 61, 65, 67, 74, 77, 104
psoralen plus UVA (PUVA), 67
psoriasis, 33, 92

Q

quality of life, viii, ix, 2, 11, 13, 14, 31, 32, 37, 38, 52, 54, 74, 79, 90, 101, 102, 103, 104, 110
quartile, 66
quaternary ammonium, 65
questionnaire, 38, 100

R

radiation, 42
rash, 12, 36, 74

reactions, 6, 9, 12, 42, 43, 57, 92, 95
reactivity, 19, 26, 28
reading, 47
recognition, vii, 1
recommendations, 107, 108
regression, 87
regression model, 87
relaxation, 32
relevance, 43, 95
reliability, 100
relief, 62, 67
remission, 12, 58
repair, 89, 109
resentment, 39
resistance, 8, 10, 62, 63, 93
resolution, 109
response, 28, 52, 55, 57, 58, 59, 60, 61, 111, 117
retardation, 53
rhinitis, 2, 81
risk, 3, 5, 13, 14, 36, 47, 48, 49, 50, 53, 59, 60, 61, 62, 67, 68, 70, 73, 75, 77, 86, 88, 89, 96, 98, 108, 115, 118
rosacea, 53

S

safety, 42, 51, 54, 57, 59, 60, 109, 110, 111, 114
saturated fatty acids, 76
scabies, 33, 34
scaling, vii, viii, 1, 21, 30, 76
school, vii, 37, 38
schooling, 31
SCORing of Atopic Dermatitis (SCORAD), viii, 14, 29
SEA, 92
seafood, 13
seborrheic dermatitis, 33
second-generation cephalosporin, 62
secrete, 9
secretion, 61
sedative, 62
selenium, 14
self-control, 118

self-esteem, 37
sensation, 37, 46, 51, 53, 55
sensitivity, 95, 107, 117
sensitization, vii, 1, 5, 14, 15, 45, 72, 87, 96, 97, 115, 117
serine, 90
serum, 6, 11, 14, 26, 30, 41, 43, 48, 92, 119
sheep, 49
shellfish, 14, 46
showing, 39
shrimp, 13
sibling, 13, 48
side effects, 53, 66, 73
signs, 29, 30, 63
silk, 64, 65, 114
silver, 64, 66, 114
Singapore, 91, 102, 118, 120
skin, vii, ix, 1, 5, 6, 7, 8, 9, 12, 14, 15, 16, 17, 19, 20, 21, 23, 25, 26, 31, 33, 34, 35, 38, 42, 43, 45, 46, 50, 51, 52, 53, 54, 56, 59, 61, 63, 64, 65, 66, 67, 72, 77, 79, 90, 91, 93, 95, 96, 97, 101, 102, 109, 111, 112, 113, 114, 118, 119
skin cancer, 59, 61, 112
skin diseases, 15, 96, 111
sleep deprivation, 61
sleep disturbance, 29, 31, 38, 103, 104
smallpox, 36, 103
smoking, 46, 96
social development, 31, 38
society, 39, 104
solvents, 27
somnolence, 62
squamous cell, 91
stabilization, 54
standardization, 43
steroids, 73
stigma, 36
stomatitis, 33
stress, ix, 2, 12, 15, 37, 39, 45, 50, 97
striae, 53, 60
structure, 90
subacute, viii, 21
Subacute lesions, viii, 21
subgroups, 98

success rate, 56
supplementation, 15, 70, 75, 76, 77, 107, 115, 118, 119
suppression, 52, 53, 60
surface area, 30, 52, 57
surface component, 9
susceptibility, 9, 88
symptoms, 4, 12, 13, 14, 20, 29, 35, 42, 43, 49, 61, 70, 72, 76, 77, 86, 87, 88, 99, 119, 120
syndrome, 36, 41, 53, 60, 103, 115
synthesis, 10, 54, 110, 120

T

T cell, 93, 101
T lymphocytes, 111
tar, 66
target, 31, 52
techniques, 9
telangiectasia, 53
testing, 42, 105, 106
textiles, 64, 65, 113, 114
TGF, 48, 107
T-helper cell, 54
therapy, ix, 42, 45, 52, 53, 58, 61, 62, 63, 64, 66, 68, 72, 74, 75, 90, 92, 93, 102, 103, 105, 109, 110, 113
thymus, 30, 41, 100
toddlers, 51
topical antibiotics, 62
toxicity, 54, 61, 73
toxin, 64
trafficking, 31
transcription, 52, 54, 109
transcription factors, 109
transforming growth factor, 48, 55, 68
transport, 91
trauma, 7
treatment, 10, 11, 31, 38, 43, 45, 52, 53, 55, 56, 57, 58, 59, 61, 62, 63, 66, 67, 68, 70, 71, 72, 73, 75, 76, 77, 78, 79, 83, 86, 87, 92, 93, 97, 99, 102, 108, 109, 110, 111, 112, 113, 114, 115, 116, 117, 118, 119, 120

tremor, 61
trial, 10, 49, 64, 68, 70, 71, 72, 74, 77, 78, 92, 93, 94, 110, 112, 113, 114, 115, 116, 117, 118, 119, 120
triggers, 62, 88
twins, 5

U

UK, ix, 118
United Kingdom, 25
United States, 3, 73, 86, 104
urban areas, 3
urea, 51, 108
urticaria, 12, 34
USA, 30, 101
uveitis, 36

V

vaccine, 103, 111
validation, 99, 101
valuation, 106
variables, 86
vasoconstriction, 67
videos, 114
viruses, 8
vitamin, 78, 119

W

warts, 36
water, 7, 8, 21, 45, 46, 51, 52, 67, 75, 89, 90, 120
weeping, viii, 21, 30
weeping lesions, viii, 21
well-being, 104
withdrawal, 54

Z

zinc, 14, 15